Forever Chemicals
How PFAS Pollutes Our Blood and Lives

Marko Vovk

Copyright © 2025 by Marko Vovk

All rights reserved.

No portion of this book may be reproduced without written permission from the publisher or author except as permitted by U.S. copyright law.

This publication is designed to provide accurate and authoritative information regarding the subject matter covered. It is sold with the understanding that neither the author nor the publisher is engaged in rendering legal.

For permissions requests: Fixyourtoxichome.com

Paperback: ISBN: 979-8-9925958-0-2
Ebook::   ISBN: 979-8-9925958-1-9

Cover Design by Marko Vovk (2nd Draft 2-21-25)

Book Edit: Non-Human: (Autocrit, Word, Addicus, Perplexity, Grammarly Plus, Book Brush, Word Art)

Interior Design by Marko Vovk   Book Cover by Marko Vovk   Images by Google, Dezgo, Marko Vovk

Final Edit by Marko Vovk (Some minor inconsistencies may exist)   Printed in USA

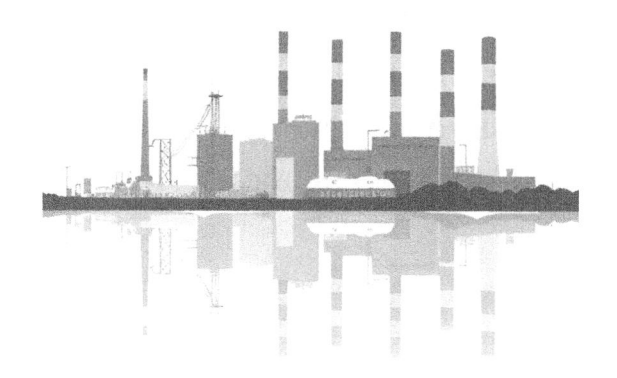

Disclaimer

This book provides general information about PFAS contamination based on available research and the author's professional experience—it does not constitute medical, legal, or environmental advice. Readers should consult qualified professionals for specific guidance. While rigorous due diligence was applied using tools like Grammarly, AutoCrit, and Perplexity, minor inconsistencies or formatting issues may exist due to the self-edited nature of this work—the author assumes no liability for adverse effects from the use or application of this content.

A revised second edition will be published in 2026 to incorporate new scientific findings, regulatory updates, reader feedback, and refinements. Corrections or suggestions may be submitted via FixYourToxicHome.com. Thank you for supporting independent publishing and the fight against "forever chemicals."

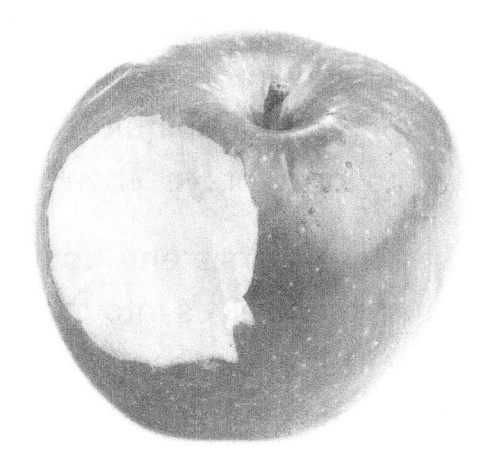

Prologue

Imagine a silent invader, creeping into every corner of your home, touching everything you eat, drink, and breathe. For 42 years, I've been on the frontlines of the battle for healthier homes, guiding countless families through the maze of visible threats like asbestos, radon, VOC's, Lead,, EMF's and mold. But as I transitioned from on-site inspections to consulting, a chilling realization dawned on me: the most insidious dangers were the ones we couldn't see.

This epiphany struck me one ordinary morning as I prepared breakfast. The scratched non-stick pan, the knife-scored paper plate, the chlorine-laced tap water - suddenly, these everyday items became sinister messengers. They whispered of a ubiquitous threat I had overlooked for far too long: forever chemicals.

Known as PFAS, these persistent pollutants have stealthily intertwined themselves into the structure of our daily lives. They lurk in our cookware, food packaging, water supplies, and countless other products we use without a second thought. As an experienced home inspector and health advocate, I was stunned to realize how blind I'd been to this pervasive danger.

This book is born from that moment of clarity - a comprehensive guide to understanding and combating the PFAS crisis that threatens our homes and health. Drawing on decades of expertise and meticulous research, I'll take you on an odyssey through your own living space, revealing the hidden sources of these chemicals and equipping you with practical strategies to protect yourself and your loved ones.

Whether you're a concerned parent, a health-conscious individual, or simply someone who wants to make informed choices about your environment, this book offers invaluable insights into a critical yet often overlooked aspect of modern living. Join me as we pull back the veil on the world of forever chemicals and embark on a mission to create truly healthier home.

Contents

Introduction	XI
1. PFAS Per- and Polyfluoroalkyl Substances.	1
2. The History of PFAS	8
3. Manufacturers of PFAS	15
4. PFAS in Our Products and in our Daily Lives	26
5. PFAS Contamination from Industry, Manufactures, Landfills, and Agriculture	40
6. The PFAS Nightmare: DuPont in Parkersburg	46
7. PFAS and Human Health	51
8. Wildlife, Birds, Fish Fisherman and Hunters	60
9. Regulations	72
10. PFAS Litigation	81
11. PFAS in Fresh Produce	89
12. So What Can We Do?	93
13. Bibligraphy	100

14. EPA Update 2025   115
15. Further Reading   118

Introduction

PFAS, or per- and Polyfluoroalkyl Substances, are a group of synthetic chemicals that have permeated our environment and daily lives. First developed in the 1950s, these compounds contain strong carbon-fluorine bonds, making them resistant to heat, water, and oil. Their unique properties led to widespread use in thousands of consumer and industrial products.

Manufacturers extract fluorine from fluorspar mines in China, Mexico, and Mongolia to create PFAS. The production process involves electrochemical fluorination or telomerization, resulting in various PFAS compounds. These chemicals persist in the environment for thousands of years, earning them the "forever chemicals.

PFAS contamination affects water, soil, air, and living organisms worldwide. Human activities release these substances through industrial processes and consumer product use. Contamination sources include manufacturing sites, firefighting foam applications, and landfills. The pollution impacts drinking water supplies and food chains globally, raising concerns about long-term health effects.

Scientists have linked PFAS exposure to numerous health issues, including cancer, thyroid disease, and immune system disorders. These chemicals bioaccumulate in the human body, potentially causing harm even at low exposure levels. The extent of PFAS-related health impacts remains unknown, prompting ongoing research and regulatory scrutiny.

The history of PFAS spans decades, with companies like 3M and DuPont playing key roles in their development and production. DuPont's accidental discovery of polytetrafluoroethylene (PTFE) in 1938 led to the creation of Teflon, revolutionizing non-stick cookware. 3M introduced Scotchgard in 1953, containing PFOS for stain resistance.

PFAS production increased throughout the 1960s and 1970s, finding applications in various industries. The U.S. Navy and 3M developed aqueous film-forming foam (AFFF) containing PFAS for firefighting purposes. This foam saw widespread use at military installations, airports, and fire departments, contributing to environmental contamination.

Early signs of PFAS toxicity emerged in the 1970s, with internal research linking these chemicals to liver damage. Despite growing concerns, production continued to expand. It wasn't until the 2000s that public awareness and regulatory action began to catch up with the scientific evidence of PFAS risks.

The environmental impact of PFAS extends beyond human health. These chemicals accumulate in wildlife, affecting various species' reproduction and survival rates. PFAS contamination has been detected in remote Arctic regions, emphasizing the global reach of this pollution. The long-term consequences for ecosystems and biodiversity remain a subject of ongoing study.

Agricultural lands are significantly contaminated with PFAS, often due to the application of biosolids from wastewater treatment plants. Farmers unknowingly spread PFAS-laden fertilizers on their fields, contaminating crops and livestock. This has resulted in devastating economic losses for some farmers and raised concerns about food safety.

The regulatory framework for PFAS continues to evolve as new information emerges. The Environmental Protection Agency (EPA) has taken steps to address PFAS contamination, including setting drinking water standards and designating certain PFAS as hazardous substances. States have implemented their restrictions, often stricter than federal guidelines.

PFAS detection and remediation present significant technical and economic hurdles. Current testing methods can be expensive and time-consuming, limiting widespread monitoring efforts. Remediation technologies for PFAS-contaminated sites are still developing, with costs often reaching millions per location.

The legal battle surrounding PFAS has intensified in recent years. Major manufacturers face thousands of lawsuits from individuals, communities, and states seeking compensation for contamination and health impacts. These legal actions have resulted in multi-million dollar settlements and increased scrutiny of corporate practices.

As research progresses, scientists uncover new information about the health effects of PFAS exposure. Studies have linked these chemicals to developmental issues, hormone disruption, and decreased vaccine response. The impact on vulnerable populations, such as pregnant women and children, is of particular concern.

This book explores the complex issue of PFAS contamination, examining its history, environmental impact, health effects, and ongoing efforts to address this global ecological crisis. Through a comprehensive analysis of scientific research, regulatory actions, and real-world case studies, we aim to provide a thorough understanding of the PFAS problem and the obstacles we face in addressing it.

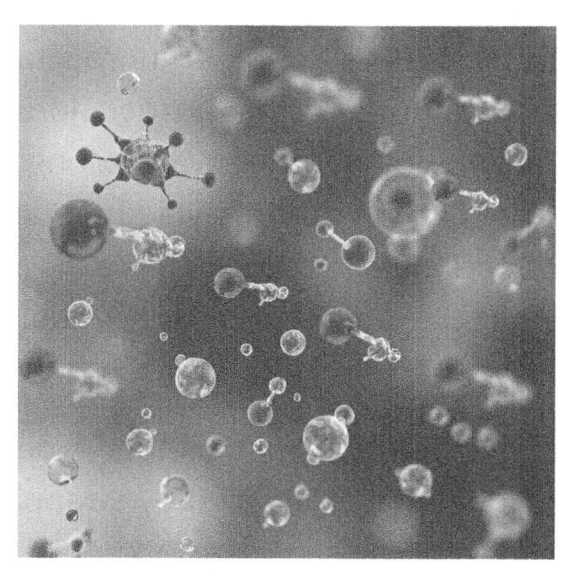

Chapter 1

PFAS Per- and Polyfluoroalkyl Substances.

PFAS stands for per- and Polyfluoroalkyl Substances. These human-made chemicals were first used in the 1950s. They contain carbon-fluorine bonds, which make them resistant to heat, water, and oil. PFAS appears in thousands of consumer and industrial products. The chemicals resist degradation and remain in the environment for thousands of years.

PFAS are synthetic chemicals with multiple fluorine atoms attached to an alkyl chain. They include perfluorooctanoic acid (PFOA) and perfluorooctanesulfonic acid (PFOS). Manufacturers extract fluorine from fluorspar mines in China, Mexico, and Mongolia. Companies transport raw materials via ships and trucks to production facilities. Factories create PFAS through electrochemical fluorination or telomerization processes.

Recently, PFOA and PFOS were banned from production. However, they were replaced by swapping chemicals. These new chemicals are also known as regrettable substitutes, making them as bad, if not worse. This situation is similar to when Bisphenol A know as BPA in plastic was changed to Bisphenol S know as BPS, which was equally harmful. Today, we have over 15,000 PFAS products, also known as "Forever Chemicals." These ubiquitous chemicals are everywhere and in the blood of 97% of all humans on earth.

> The following section contains technical information, while the rest of the book maintains an easy-to-read style. Electrochemical fluorination (ECF) disperses organic feedstocks in liquid anhydrous hydrogen fluoride. An electric current passes through the solution, replacing hydrogen atoms with fluorine. This

> process fragments and rearranges the carbon skeleton. ECF produces linear and branched perfluorinated isomers.
>
> Telomerization reacts perfluoroalkyl iodides with tetrafluoroethylene, resulting in even-numbered carbon chain lengths with an iodide functional end group. I could devote an entire chapter to the chemical properties and manufacturing processes, but I won't because this is not an engineering book. For the sake of simplicity, we will use the term PFAS along with "Forever Chemicals" because there are too many varieties. For the average reader, we don't need to jump into specifics. We want to know the facts and what we can do about them. So, for the remainder of this book, we will keep it simple.

Scientists call PFAS "forever chemicals" because they persist in the environment. Because of their strong carbon-fluorine bonds, these substances resist degradation. Over time, PFAS accumulate in organisms and ecosystems, and they remain stable under extreme conditions like high temperatures.

I know some are nodding their heads because I used the word fluorine. Yes, it's the same fluoride some countries put in water to help keep our teeth from decay. I'm not going to get into the whole fluoride issue, but I can say one thing: our bodies don't need fluoride. We get more fluoride from many PFAS principal water treatment plants. Most of the world does not put fluoride into drinking water. These strong carbon-fluorine bonds cannot be broken down unless we have extreme heat and persist for centuries.

Their longevity poses difficulties for removal efforts. PFAS can remain in the environment for up to 1,000 years after use. PFAS contamination affects water, soil, air, and organisms worldwide. These chemicals appear in remote locations, including Arctic regions and deep oceans. Human activities release PFAS through industrial processes and consumer product use. Contamination sources include manufacturing sites, firefighting foam applications, and landfills. PFAS pollution impacts drinking water supplies and food chains globally.

Perfluorooctanoic acid (PFOA) and perfluorobutane sulfonic acid (PFOS), once used in various consumer products, have been phased out due to health concerns. However, they've been replaced by chemicals like GenX (hexafluoropropylene oxide dimer acid) and other short-chain PFAS compounds. Contrary to industry claims of improved safety, recent studies suggest these replacements may be equally harmful or more detrimental than their predecessors.

A 2023 study published in the Chemical Engineering Journal found that short-chain PFAS are "more widely detected, more persistent and mobile in aquatic systems. This poses more risks to human and ecosystem health" than long-chain PFAS like PFOA and PFOS.

Alarmingly, chemical manufacturers have been aware of the potential dangers of these substances since the 1970s. Internal documents from companies like 3M and DuPont reveal early knowledge of their toxicity and environmental persistence.

The PFAS industry's tactics resemble those employed by tobacco companies, which concealed the health risks of smoking for decades. It wasn't until the late 1990s that tobacco executives admitted under oath their products caused cancer and were addictive. The nuclear industry demonstrated a cavalier attitude towards public safety in the 1950s when companies like the A.C. Gilbert Company marketed radioactive "Atomic Energy Lab" kits to children as educational toys.

These kits, which contained actual uranium ore samples and various radioactive sources, were sold from 1950 to 1951 before being discontinued. As history repeats itself with PFAS, we see a familiar pattern of corporate deception, concealment of scientific evidence, and disregard for public health.

With all this industrial pollution contaminating our lands and water, we face major unintended consequences and significant collateral damage.

In the plant and animal kingdoms, plants uptake PFAS from contaminated soil and water, influenced by factors like soil concentration, organic matter, pH, and mineral surfaces. Due to their stronger sorption into soil and roots, Long-chain PFAS have low plant transfer factors. They're less likely to move from soil to plant tissues and above-ground parts, and this transfer rate decreases with increasing PFAS chain length. PFAS also accumulates in wildlife, causing health effects and abnormalities.

Studies show that PFAS exposure in animals suppresses immunity, damages the liver, and leads to developmental and reproductive issues. Aquatic birds like Double-crested Cormorants and Little Ringed Plovers have experienced reduced hatching success due to PFAS exposure. PFAS has been detected in diverse bird species globally, including northern cardinals in Hawaii, Snow Buntings in the Arctic, and American Flamingos in the Caribbean. Effects in birds often mirror those in humans, making avian studies useful indicators of broader wildlife and public health risks.

While we will jump into the effects on humans later, let's first explore some historical context to understand the origins and development of PFAS better.

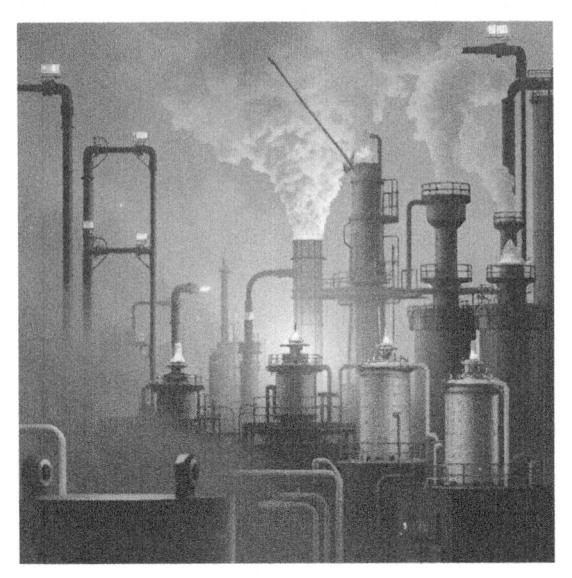

Chapter 2

The History of PFAS

PFAS emerged in the 1930s when scientists discovered the unique properties of fluorine-carbon bonds. Roy Plunkett accidentally created polytetrafluoroethylene (PTFE) while working at DuPont in 1938, leading to Teflon, a non-stick coating with numerous applications. One of the earliest significant uses of PFAS was in the Manhattan Project during World War

II, where PTFE played an essential role in the development of the atomic bomb.

It was used in uranium enrichment, serving in gaskets and valves to contain corrosive gases, and also functioned as a fire suppressant, coolant, and lubricant in nuclear processes. In my book "Nuclear Extinction Event is Killing Our Families," I discuss how the nuclear industry, much like the PFAS industry, is having a devastating impact on our planet and its inhabitants.

In 1945, DuPont trademarked PTFE as Teflon, marking the beginning of commercial PFAS production. 3M acquired the Simons Process that same year, enabling large-scale fluorochemical manufacturing. The 1950s saw a rapid expansion of PFAS use in consumer products. As we explore in later chapters, these industrial plants contaminated surrounding areas and polluted water sources. In 1953, 3M introduced Scotchgard, which contains perfluorobutane sulfonic acid (PFOS). PFAS production increased throughout the 1960s and 1970s. Little did the public know these treated carpets would contaminate the bloodstreams of the occupants.

3M and the U.S. Navy developed aqueous film-forming foam (AFF) and aqueous Film-Forming Foam containing PFOS and PFOA. Military sites, airports, and firefighting centers adopted AFFF worldwide and sprayed it on runways and in forests. Little did they know the runoff would contaminate wells, aquifers, and ecosystems. PFAS found applications in the aerospace, automotive, construction, and electronics industries. That new car smell was not a breath of fresh air, and the leather or fabric coatings released particles that entered our bodies.

Consumer products containing these chemicals, like non-stick cookware and water-repellent clothing, gained widespread popularity. However, these convenient items came with hidden risks. When scratched by cooking utensils, non-stick pans could release PFAS particles into meals. Similarly, washing our treated clothing sent PFAS-contaminated water to treatment plants ill-equipped to remove these persistent chemicals.

In 1969, Gore-Tex, another PFAS-containing product, was invented, further expanding the use of PFAS in consumer goods. This innovation led to a proliferation of PFAS-treated products, including waterproof jackets and outdoor gear, stain-resistant carpets and upholstery, grease-resistant food packaging, firefighting foam, and certain cosmetics and personal care products.

The widespread adoption of these products exposed consumers to harmful chemicals, emphasizing the need for greater awareness and regulation of PFAS in everyday items. Early signs of PFAS toxicity emerged in the 1970s and 1980s.

3M's internal research linked PFOA and PFOS to liver damage. In 1981, a study by 3M found PFAS in the blood of its workers, raising issues about occupational exposure. Aware of potential risks, some manufacturers took precautionary measures by relocating women of childbearing age to other parts of their factories.

This decision was driven by knowledge of PFAS-related issues such as low birth weights, complications with breastfeeding, and fetal development problems, topics we will explore in greater detail in later chapters.

Despite these alarming findings, PFAS production continued to grow. Companies expanded product lines and explored new applications driven by the chemicals' persistence and effectiveness. PFAS became integral to many industrial processes and consumer goods, leading to widespread adoption across various sectors.

Environmental contamination from PFAS manufacturing and use became evident in the 1980s and 1990s. Researchers detected PFAS in wildlife and human blood samples, revealing the chemicals' widespread presence and bioaccumulation potential. Studies began to uncover health risks associated with PFAS exposure. While industry knowledge of PFAS hazards grew, public awareness remained limited. Today, as you read this book, only about 30% of the population has heard of "Forever Chemicals" beyond the well-publicized issues with Teflon. Many people are unaware these substances are ubiquitous and present in numerous products beyond their frying pans.

Regulatory agencies began investigating PFAS impacts in the early 2000s, marking a regulation and public awareness shift. In 2000, 3M announced a voluntary phase-out of PFOA and PFOS production due to growing health concerns. In 2006, the EPA launched the PFOA Stewardship Program, aiming to reduce emissions and product content of PFOA and related chemicals by 95% by 2010 and eliminate them by 2015.

Companies adopted improved manufacturing processes and filtration systems to meet these goals. However, many alternative chemicals introduced were later found to be as harmful. As evidence of PFAS health risks grew, regulators increased oversight. In 2009, the EPA issued provisional health advisories for PFOA and PFOS in drinking water. By 2016, these were updated to lifetime health advisories set at 70 parts per trillion.

In 2020, the EPA strengthened regulations requiring notice and review before phased-out long-chain PFAS could be reintroduced. These actions reflected mounting concerns about the widespread contamination and potential health impacts of PFAS exposure. The Stockholm Convention on Persistent Organic Pollutants took significant international action against PFAS.

In 2009, it added PFOS, its salts, and perfluorooctane sulfonyl fluoride (PFOSF) to Annex B, restricting their production and use globally. The treaty requires countries to reduce or eliminate the release of listed pollutants, promote best practices to prevent contamination and manage waste containing these chemicals.

As we move forward in history, a significant milestone occurred in 2016 when the EPA established a lifetime health advisory for PFOA and PFOS in drinking water at 70 parts per trillion. To put this in perspective, 70 parts per trillion is equivalent to about one drop of water in 20 Olympic-sized swimming pools, demonstrating the potency of these chemicals.

This minuscule amount shows the severe toxicity of PFAS. In 2019, the EPA released the PFAS Action Plan, outlining a comprehensive approach to addressing contamination. This plan included steps to evaluate the need for a maximum contaminant level for PFOA and PFOS, consider designating PFAS as hazardous substances, and develop groundwater cleanup recommendations.

Congress passed legislation requiring PFAS monitoring and cleanup at military sites through the National Defense Authorization Act. This legislation mandated the Department of Defense to phase out the use of PFAS-containing firefighting foam, provide blood testing for military firefighters, and enter into cooperative agreements with communities for testing, monitoring, and cleanup of PFAS contamination.

Lawsuits against PFAS manufacturers and users have proliferated, seeking compensation for environmental and health impacts, which we will explore in more detail later. Many states are implementing their PFAS regulations, which are often more stringent than federal guidelines. These state-level actions reflect growing public concern and the need for more comprehensive protection against PFAS contamination.

Now that we have a brief overview of history, let's examine the key players in the PFAS saga.

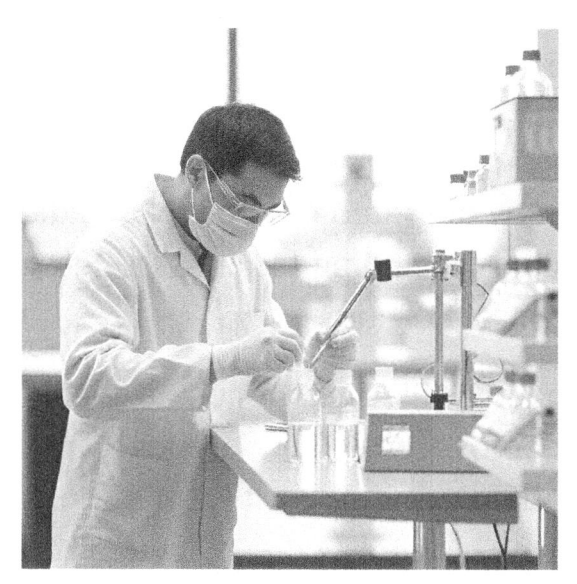

Chapter 3

Manufacturers of PFAS

PFAS emerged as a revolutionary class of chemicals in the mid-20th century, with several manufacturers becoming key players in the industry. 3M Company pioneered PFAS production, developing compounds like PFOS (perfluorooctane sulfonic acid) and PFOA (perfluorooctanoic acid). In 1953, 3M introduced Scotchgard, a stain-resistant product containing PFOS, which gained popularity in consumer and industrial markets.

3M's PFAS production was substantial, with its Cottage Grove facility in Minnesota serving as the primary manufacturing site. By the 1990s, 3M produced millions of pounds of PFOS annually, with global sales of PFOS-based products reaching $300 million annually. The company operated multiple plants dedicated to PFAS production, including facilities in Decatur, Alabama, and Antwerp, Belgium.

As 3M expanded its PFAS portfolio, the chemicals found applications across various industries. One significant use was firefighting foam, with 3M supplying Aqueous Film-Forming Foam (AFFF) to military and civilian users. AFFF was employed in numerous large-scale fire incidents, including aircraft crashes and fuel storage fires. While not typically used for forest fires, AFFF was deployed in industrial accidents and at military bases for training exercises.

Several incidents in which AFFF was used include the USS Forrestal fire in 1967, which claimed 134 lives and prompted the widespread adoption of AFFF in the US Navy. The foam was also used at airports and refineries worldwide. However, this wide spread use led to environmental contamination, with PFAS from firefighting foam seeping into groundwater and soil at many sites worldwide.

DuPont entered the PFAS market in 1938 when it discovered polytetrafluoroethylene (PTFE) at its Jackson Laboratory in Deepwater, New Jersey. Chemist Roy J. Plunkett found the substance while working on refrigerant chemicals. 1945, the company trademarked PTFE as Teflon, revolutionizing nonstick cookware and numerous other industries.

DuPont's Washington Works plant in Parkersburg, West Virginia, became a significant hub for PFAS production. The facility began manufacturing Teflon and other fluoropolymers in 1951 and continued for decades. As production expanded, environmental concerns grew as PFAS contamination spread from the plant into surrounding communities and waterways.

While Washington Works was a significant PFAS production site, DuPont operated other facilities globally. The company's Dordrecht Works in the Netherlands and its Changshu plant in China also produced PFAS chemicals. DuPont's Chambers Works in Deepwater, New Jersey, and its Fayetteville Works in North Carolina were additional PFAS manufacturing locations in the United States.

Other companies also entered the PFAS market. 3M began producing PFAS in 1949 at its Cottage Grove facility in Minnesota, becoming a major competitor to

DuPont. In Japan, Daikin Industries started PFAS production in the 1970s. European companies like Solvay in Belgium and Arkema in France also became large PFAS manufacturers.

As awareness of PFAS-related health and environmental risks grew, regulatory scrutiny intensified. In 2006, the EPA launched the PFOA Stewardship Program, prompting major manufacturers to phase out certain PFAS chemicals. This led to industry shifts, with some companies developing alternative PFAS formulations while others exited the market.

Chemours spun off DuPont in 2015, inheriting the PFAS business centered at the Washington Works plant in Parkersburg, West Virginia. The new company continued producing fluoropolymers and other PFAS compounds used in various applications, including nonstick, water-repellent clothing, food packaging, and firefighting foam.

Chemours developed GenX as a replacement for PFOA, but it faces scrutiny over its safety. While both are part of the PFAS family, GenX has a shorter carbon chain (six carbon atoms) than PFOA's (eight carbon atoms), making it less persistent in the environment. However, studies have shown that GenX may be equally harmful or more toxic than PFOA.

Corteva emerged as another DuPont spinoff in 2019. The company focuses on agricultural chemicals and produces seeds, crop protection products, and digital solutions for farmers. Corteva operates globally, with a significant presence in North America, Europe, Latin America, and Asia Pacific. Key products include corn and soybean seeds, herbicides, and insecticides.

Corteva inherited some PFAS liabilities from its parent corporation. For example, it assumed responsibility for certain environmental cleanup costs and potential legal claims related to historical PFAS contamination at various sites. These liabilities include groundwater contamination issues and ongoing litigation related to PFAS exposure in communities near former DuPont facilities.

Other PFAS producers include Arkema, BASF, and Daikin, each with a global presence and specialized product lines. These companies manufacture a range of fluoropolymers and fluorosurfactants in various industries.

Arkema, headquartered in Colombes, France, produces polyvinylidene fluoride (PVDF) for industrial applications. PVDF is a nonreactive thermoplastic fluoropolymer known for its strength, flexibility, and resistance to solvents, acids, and heat. It is marketed under the Kynar brand and used in chemical processing equipment, lithium-ion batteries, and architectural coatings. The company has production facilities in Pierre-Bénite, France, and Changshu, China.

BASF, based in Ludwigshafen, Germany, focuses on fluorinated polymers for various sectors. Their product portfolio includes fluoroelastomers and fluorosurfactants used in the automotive, electronics, and construction industries. BASF operates PFAS production sites in Ludwigshafen, Germany; Antwerp, Belgium; Geismar, USA; and Nanjing, China. Their fluoropolymers are utilized in fuel hoses, O-rings, and electrical insulation.

Daikin, headquartered in Osaka, Japan, specializes in refrigerants and PFAS coatings. PFAS, per- and polyfluoroalkyl substances, is a group of man-made chemicals, including PTFE, PVDF, and other fluoropolymers. Daikin produces refrigerants like R-32, a hydrofluorocarbon used in air conditioning systems. Their PFAS-based coatings, such as the Optool line, are used for surface treatments in electronics and automotive applications. Daikin's products are semiconductors, printed circuit boards, and automotive sensors.

These PFAS products are integral to semiconductors, circuit boards, and high-performance wiring insulation. Manufacturing electronics fans are also found in fuel system components, lubricants, and sensors for advanced driver assistance systems in the automotive sector. In construction, PFAS-based materials are used in weather-resistant architectural coatings, sealants, and high-performance insulation.

Closed PFAS manufacturing facilities have left a toxic legacy of contamination across the United States. Some examples include the 3M Cottage Grove plant in Minnesota, DuPont's Chambers Works in New Jersey, and the Saint-Gobain Performance Plastics site in Hoosick Falls, New York. These sites have caused extensive soil, groundwater, and surface water contamination, which we will explore later in the book.

Minnesota's 3M Cottage Grove plant ceased PFAS production in 2002, but its environmental impact persists. Groundwater contamination at the site has affected an area of more than 150 square miles, impacting the drinking water supplies of over 140,000 Minnesotans. Ongoing remediation efforts include groundwater treatment and soil excavation, with costs estimated to be hundreds of millions of dollars.

DuPont's Chambers Works in New Jersey faces similar obstacles after decades of PFAS manufacturing. The site has been pumping and treating groundwater since the 1970s, with PFOA and other "Teflon chemicals" appearing in local water health tests at levels exceeding state safety standards. The cleanup efforts at Chambers Works exemplify the complex nature of addressing PFAS contamination at Superfund sites.

Superfund sites, designated under the Comprehensive Environmental Response, Compensation, and Liability Act (CERCLA), show the long-term consequences of PFAS production. These sites are among the nation's most contaminated areas, requiring extensive, federally overseen cleanup processes. The Saint-Gobain Performance Plastics site in Hoosick Falls, New York, is one such example. PFOA from the facility seeped into groundwater, contaminating local water supplies and affecting residents' health. The EPA's Superfund designation has initiated a complex cleanup process, with investigations revealing widespread PFAS contamination in the surrounding area.

The Washington Works plant in West Virginia, now owned by Chemours, has become another notorious Superfund site. DuPont's long-standing PFAS production contaminated the Ohio River Valley, leading to thousands of residents filing lawsuits over health impacts. This case resulted in a landmark settlement and increased scrutiny of PFAS. Cleanup efforts continue, addressing decades of environmental damage. Recent agreements require Chemours to conduct extensive sampling for PFAS contamination surrounding the facility, reflecting the ongoing remediation obstacles .

Global PFAS production continues despite growing scrutiny. Manufacturers in China and other countries are expanding operations, filling the void left by stricter regulations in Western nations. For instance, in recent years, Shandong Dongyue Group, one of China's largest fluorochemical producers, has increased its PFAS production capacity. Similarly, Indian company Gujarat Fluorochemicals Limited has expanded its fluoropolymer manufacturing facilities. International regulations lag behind those in the United States and Europe.

While the EU and US have implemented stricter controls, many developing countries have yet to establish comprehensive PFAS regulations. For example, as of 2024, China had only restricted a handful of PFAS compounds, focusing on PFOS and its derivatives. We will explore global regulatory disparities in greater detail later in the book. The economic impact of PFAS litigation and regulation is changing the industry. Companies are setting aside billions for potential settlements and cleanup costs.

Some are considering exiting the PFAS market altogether. In 2022, 3M announced its intention to phase out PFAS production by 2025, citing regulatory pressures and changing market dynamics. Chemours, a DuPont spinoff, also faced significant financial pressure due to PFAS-related liabilities. Other companies are doubling down on developing new PFAS compounds and betting on their ability to create safer alternatives. The economic stakes are driving research into PFAS alternatives and remediation technologies. Let's look at a partial list of major PFAS-producing companies, from largest to smallest:

1. 3M Company (USA)

2. Chemours (USA)

3. Daikin Industries (Japan)

4. Solvay (Belgium)

5. Arkema (France)

6. AGC Inc. (Japan)

7. Dongyue Group (China)

8. Gujarat Fluorochemicals (India)

9. Fluoryx (USA)

10. Merck KGaA (Germany)

This list represents only a fraction of the global PFAS industry, emphasizing its scale and complexity. Public awareness of PFAS risks is growing, influencing consumer behavior. Demand for PFAS-free products is increasing across various sectors, from cookware to clothing. Manufacturers are responding by reformulating products to eliminate PFAS, creating new market opportunities for alternative technologies. However, the transition from PFAS presents technical and economic hurdles for many industries, as these chemicals often provide unique performance characteristics that are difficult to replicate.

Now that we have considered the industry's major players, the next chapter will examine the products and how consumers use them.

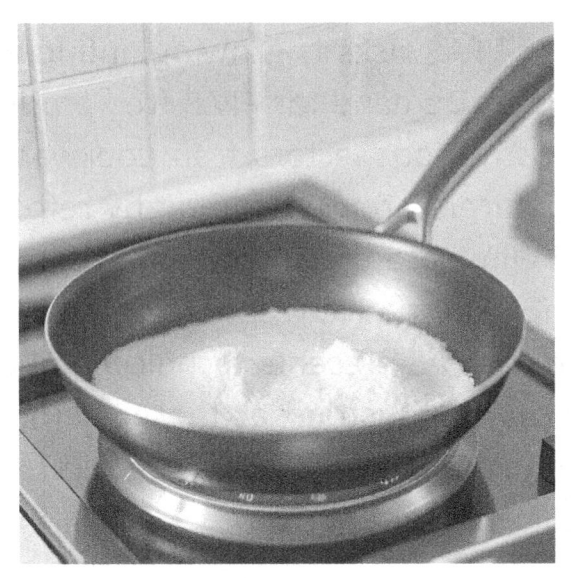

Chapter 4

PFAS in Our Products and in our Daily Lives

P FAS chemicals are pervasive in many everyday products that directly contact our skin. These chemicals make water-, grease-, and stain-repellent coatings for various consumer goods and industrial applications. Typical items include cosmetics and personal care products, water-resistant clothing and fabrics, non-stick cookware, and stain-resistant carpets and furniture.

Recent studies have shown that PFAS can be absorbed through human skin, contrary to previous beliefs that the skin acts as an effective barrier. Using 3D models of lab-grown human skin tissue, researchers found that many PFAS compounds can indeed penetrate the skin and enter the body. Shorter-chain PFAS molecules are more readily absorbed through the skin than longer-chain ones.

Animal studies have shown that PFAS absorption through the skin can cause immunosuppressive effects, including reduced antibody levels and decreased spleen and thymus weights. In humans, low-level PFAS exposure has been linked to harm to the immune system in both children and adults.

When we wash these PFAS-containing products or ourselves after using them, the chemicals end up in our wastewater. Traditional wastewater treatment plants are not designed to remove PFAS compounds. Due to their water solubility, PFAS bypass most filters in treatment facilities.

While some PFAS can be removed via biosolids or filtered out by activated carbon and certain membrane filters, these processes do not destroy the chemicals, allowing them to contaminate other parts of the environment.

Conventional wastewater treatment processes, such as activated sludge and sedimentation, are ineffective at removing PFAS. This inadequate treatment releases PFAS into receiving waters, harming aquatic ecosystems and wildlife.

The persistence of PFAS in our environment and their ability to accumulate in our bodies over time show the importance of finding more effective ways to remove these "forever" chemicals from our water systems and reduce their use in consumer products.

Food packaging incorporates PFAS to create a barrier against grease and moisture. These chemicals form a protective coating on paper and paperboard, preventing oil and water from seeping. Fast food wrappers, microwave popcorn bags, and pizza boxes utilize PFAS for their repellent properties.

When a microwave popcorn bag heats, PFAS migrates into the oil and kernels. The high temperature causes these chemicals to vaporize and coat the popcorn. Pizza boxes transfer PFAS to the pizza through direct contact with the greasy surface. Wrappers release PFAS into food through friction and heat exposure.

Candy bars and gum packaging also contain PFAS. These chemicals leach into the products during storage and transportation. A 2017 study detects PFAS in one-third of food packaging samples tested. The research examines restaurants' fast food containers, bakery bags, and beverage cups.

Consumers ingest PFAS through contaminated food and beverages. These chemicals enter the bloodstream and accumulate in organs like the liver and kidneys. They persist in the body for years, causing long-term health effects. The FDA approves certain PFAS for food-contact applications. However, growing evidence links PFAS exposure to health issues such as cancer, thyroid problems, and immune system dysfunction. Regulatory agencies face pressure to reevaluate the safety of these chemicals in food packaging.

Textiles treated with PFAS repel water, oil, and stains, making them useful in outdoor gear. Brands like Patagonia, The North Face, and Columbia incorporate PFAS into jackets, pants, and boots. Gore-Tex, a popular waterproof membrane, uses PFAS to achieve its water-resistant properties. Camping gear such as tents and sleeping bags also contain PFAS, which can directly contact the skin during use. This prolonged exposure raises concerns, as PFAS are mobile and can be absorbed through the skin, accumulating in the body over time.

PFAS-treated fabrics are also found in furniture, carpets, and automotive upholstery. Companies like Scotchgard, Stainmaster, and Sunbrella use these chemicals in products such as La-Z-Boy recliners, Mohawk carpets, and Ford vehicle seats. Babies and pets on treated carpets face increased exposure to PFAS chemicals, which can transfer through direct contact or inhalation of particles. In vehicles, seat covers, floor mats, and steering wheel covers often contain PFAS treatments.

The new car smell results from chemicals like PFAS off-gassing from interior surfaces. The global market for waterproof textiles is projected to reach $23.9 billion by 2025. However, PFAS treatments release volatile organic compounds (VOCs), which are gases emitted from treated materials. These VOCs contribute to indoor air pollution and may pose health risks over time. Prolonged exposure to PFAS-treated car interiors or home furnishings increases the likelihood of chemical accumulation in the body.

PFAS persists in the environment and bioaccumulates in human organs such as the liver and kidneys. Studies have detected these chemicals in blood samples worldwide. Some companies now offer alternatives to PFAS-treated outdoor gear. For example, Lucky Sheep produces wool and cotton sleeping bags treated with beeswax as a natural water repellent. These options provide safer choices for consumers concerned about PFAS exposure.

Firefighting foam containing PFAS, known as aqueous film-forming foam (AFF), has been widely used since the 1960s. AFFF has been effective in significant incidents like the 1986 Dupont Plaza Hotel fire in Puerto Rico and the 2018 Camp Fire in California. The foam enters soil, water, creeks, streams, and rivers, contaminating farmlands and properties.

If firefighting foam isn't cleaned up, PFAS can evaporate into the air or seep into the soil, contaminating groundwater and drinking water. In 2014, PFAS from AFFF contaminated farmland near Fairchild Air Force Base in Washington, forcing farmers to stop selling crops.

The U.S. Navy develops AFFF with 3M Corporation to combat shipboard fires. , AFFF contained perfluorooctanesulfonic acid (PFOS) or perfluorooctanoic acid (PFOA). Because of their persistence in the environment, they don't break down and will remain in the environment virtually permanently. The well-documented health effects of these two specific chemicals are being phased out in the U.S. Still, these chemicals remain present in the bodies of most Americans and our water, soil, and air.

While effective, they are also a significant source of PFAS pollution in California and worldwide. While this problem and the development of safer alternatives have led many parts of the world to restrict or eliminate AFFF. Several US States with outdated fire regulations for military installations and airports have contaminated the water of nearby communities. Once PFAS are released into the environment, they are difficult to clean up because they easily dissolve in water. These contaminants will then contaminate groundwater and drinking water.

They do not break down and build up in the environment over time, and there is no natural way to remove them, which may increase our risk of exposure to PFAS for hundreds or thousands of years.

Cosmetics and personal care products often contain PFAS to enhance durability and texture. A recent study found that PFAS was present in over half of cosmetics tested, including lipstick, foundation, and mascara.

Popular L'Oreal, Maybelline, and CoverGirl may use PFAS in their products. Lipstick, foundation, and mascara containing PFAS can enter the body through skin absorption and ingestion. Lipstick wearers may consume several pounds of product over their lifetime. PFAS in these products can be absorbed through the lips and mouth, entering the bloodstream,

Sunscreens, shampoos, and dental floss also contain PFAS. These chemicals can enter the body through skin absorption and oral exposure.

"Women use multiple personal care products daily, exposing themselves to various PFAS sources. Most are unaware of this exposure, as PFAS are often unlisted ingredients. Studies show women who use these products have higher PFAS levels in their bodies.

Women of childbearing age using PFAS-containing products risk exposing their fetuses and breastfeeding infants to these chemicals. PFAS can cross the placental barrier and accumulate in breast milk. This early-life exposure may lead to long-term health effects, which we'll explore in later chapters.

Industrial applications of PFAS span numerous sectors, including aerospace, automotive, and electronics. Factory workers handling these chemicals face significant exposure risks through inhalation, skin contact, and ingestion. Studies show workers in PFAS-related industries, such as fluorochemical plants and ski wax technicians, have elevated PFAS levels in their blood decades after exposure. These workers often report health issues like liver damage, autoimmune disorders, and cancer.

In aerospace, companies like Boeing and Airbus use PFAS in hydraulic fluids and wire insulation to prevent fires and corrosion. Hydraulic fluid leaks during maintenance or accidents release PFAS into the environment, contaminating soil and water sources. Workers exposed to these fluids risk absorbing PFAS through their skin or inhaling airborne particles during routine operations.

Automotive manufacturers such as Ford and Toyota incorporate PFAS into fuel systems, lubricants, and seals to ensure durability under extreme conditions. When fuel systems leak or lubricants are improperly disposed of, PFAS enter waterways through runoff. These chemicals contaminate aquatic ecosystems, affecting insects, fish, and other animals that rely on these habitats. Over time, this contamination spreads to drinking water supplies.

Electronics giants like Apple and Samsung use PFAS in semiconductor production and circuit board coatings to enhance performance and reliability. However, the manufacturing process releases PFAS into wastewater systems, which cannot often filter out these persistent chemicals. This pollution affects surrounding communities by contaminating local water sources and agricultural land.

Despite growing environmental concerns, PFAS remain used due to their unique properties and lack of viable alternatives. However, their persistence in the environment and harmful effects on workers, wildlife, and ecosystems show the urgent need for stricter regulations and safer substitutes.

PFAS are processing aids in plastics and rubber manufacturing, improving product quality and production efficiency. These chemicals are used in products like automotive fuel hoses, gaskets, seals, medical devices such as catheters, and surgical tubing. Companies like DuPont and 3M manufacture PFAS-based additives to enhance these applications.

PFAS improves flow and reduces defects in polymer production by minimizing friction and preventing melt fracture, which occurs when polymers break or crack during extrusion. This allows manufacturers to produce smoother, more uniform items like films for food packaging, pipes, and wires. These additives also enable faster production speeds and reduced waste, making them essential in industrial processes. Due to regulatory pressure, plastic additive makers are developing PFAS-free alternatives.

Companies like Tosaf and Clariant have introduced PFAS-free processing aids for food-contact applications, including cast and blown films. However, these alternatives carry environmental risks. Some that rely on biopolymers or other synthetic materials may still harm ecosystems or require significant energy to produce.

PFAS also finds applications in paints, adhesives, and sealants in the construction and manufacturing industries. These chemicals are incorporated into building materials like roofing membranes, paints, sealants, and solar panel glass. When it rains, PFAS from these materials wash into the soil below, contaminating groundwater. Despite their environmental impact, companies like Sherwin-Williams and 3M continue to produce PFAS-containing products. Sherwin-Williams previously faced criticism for lead-based paint that was causing many health problems.

PFAS enter drinking water through various industrial releases. Factories discharge PFAS into nearby water sources during production processes or through air emissions that settle into soil and waterways. Sewage treatment plants also release PFAS-laden effluent because they cannot filter these chemicals. Farmers across the globe have applied contaminated sludge as fertilizer on their fields, spreading PFAS into crops and livestock—a topic explored further in later chapters. Leaching from landfills has created cancer cluster zones near waste sites, where communities face elevated health risks.

People living near manufacturing facilities or construction sites face heightened exposure to PFAS through contaminated water, air, and soil. These areas often experience cancer clusters due to prolonged contact with these persistent chemicals. The widespread use PFAS is a processing aid in plastics and rubber manufacturing, improving product quality and production efficiency. These chemicals appear in food packaging, automotive parts, and medical devices. (Add in what auto parts and medical devices are needed.

PFAS improves flow and reduces defects in polymer production by lowering friction and preventing melt fracture. This allows manufacturers to create smoother, more uniform products with fewer imperfections. The chemicals enable faster production speeds and reduce waste, making them valuable in industrial processes.

Oil and gas industries use PFAS in drilling fluids and foam stimulation to enhance performance. These chemicals are injected into natural gas and oil wells as part of fracking operations. PFAS improves the stability and effectiveness of fracking fluids, helping to fracture underground formations and extract trapped oil or gas.

When PFAS-containing fracking fluids are injected into wells, they can contaminate groundwater and surface water. These chemicals may also become airborne when wells are flared or vented, exposing nearby communities. In some areas, homes and businesses are located within a few hundred feet of gas wells, increasing the risk of PFAS exposure through air and water.

Exxon Mobil and Chevron incorporate PFAS to enhance oil recovery, using these chemicals to improve the efficiency of extracting oil from underground reservoirs. The PFAS act as surfactants, reducing surface tension and allowing oil to flow more easily through rock formations. However, this practice leads to environmental contamination.

The disposal of PFAS-contaminated wastewater from fracking operations poses additional risks. Standard disposal methods include underground injection, land application, and road spreading for dust suppression or de-icing. These practices can further spread PFAS contamination to soil and water resources. In the mining industry, PFAS-containing surfactants separate minerals from ore. Miners may be exposed to these chemicals through skin contact, inhalation, or accidental ingestion. PFAS can also contaminate runoff from mining sites, affecting nearby water sources and ecosystems.

The renewable energy sector faces its own PFAS obstacles. Photovoltaic panel production involves PFAS in anti-reflective coatings and encapsulants. Solar companies use these chemicals to enhance panel efficiency and durability. However, this creates future problems about the long-term environmental impacts of disposing of solar panels at the end of their life.

As we've seen, PFAS contamination is widespread across various industries. The following chapters will explore how these chemicals will forever impact agriculture and illustrate the far-reaching consequences of PFAS use in industrial applications.

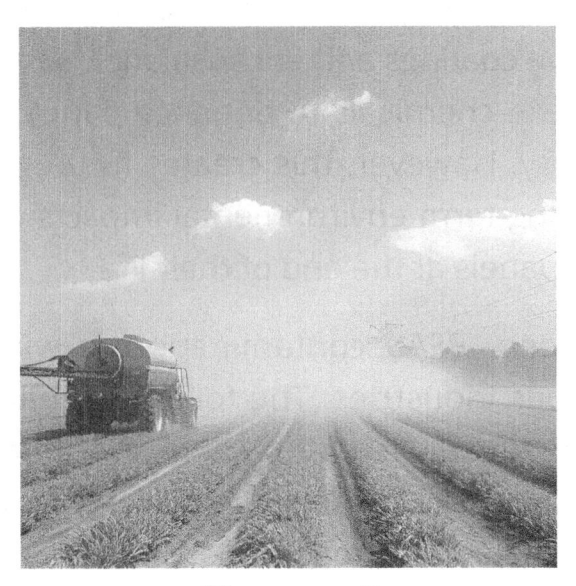

Chapter 5

PFAS Contamination from Industry, Manufactures, Landfills, and Agriculture

P FSA waste comes from manufacturing, consumer goods, and industrial uses in China, the USA, and Europe. Companies dispose of PFAS through incineration, landfilling, and deep well injection. These methods contribute to environmental contamination through air emissions, groundwater leaching, and underground migration.

Incineration burns PFAS at temperatures above 1000°C in US and European facilities. Landfills store PFAS-containing waste, which can leach into groundwater over decades. Most landfills do not test for PFAS contamination. The US has about 3,000 active landfills covering 250,000 acres.

Thousands of unregulated dump sites exist in forests, farms, and other areas, which pose additional contamination risks. Deep well injection pumps PFAS waste into underground formations, isolating contaminants. This method is used in states like Texas and Ohio.

Deep well injection has long-term risks, including potential groundwater contamination. PFAS can migrate through geological formations over time, and the full environmental impact of this disposal method remains uncertain.

PFAS contamination from landfills poses a significant environmental and health risk. Leachate, the liquid filtering through landfill waste, often contains high PFAS levels. A 2020 study revealed PFAS concentrations in landfill leachate (93,100 ppt) far exceeded those in wastewater treatment plants. Various waste types contribute to PFAS in landfills.

A 2023 study found that municipal solid waste leachate contained the highest PFAS levels (10,000 ppt), followed by construction debris (6,200 ppt) and incineration ash (1,300 ppt). These levels exceed the EPA's proposed guidelines of 4 ppt by 250,000%, 155,000%, and 32,500%. Contaminated leachate often enters municipal wastewater treatment plants, which struggle to remove PFAS. The EPA's old guideline for PFOA and PFOS combined was 70 ppt.

New guidelines propose four PPTs for each compound, emphasizing increased concern. The industrial discharge also contributes to PFAS water contamination. In New Jersey, drinking water PFAS levels reached 1,360 ppt for PFOA and 2,790 ppt for PFHxS, exceeding safety standards by 34,000% and 69,750%. Communities near contaminated sites face disproportionate risks. A 2023 study found that 25% of the population in 18 states received water with PFAS levels above five ppt, 25% higher than new guidelines. Minority communities often face higher exposure rates, raising environmental justice concerns.

Wastewater treatment plants receive PFAS from industrial and residential sources. The treatment removes 10-50% of PFAS, discharging 95% of treated wastewater into water resources. The remaining 5% becomes sludge, which facilities convert into biosolids for land application. Conventional methods fail to remove PFAS from sewage. Biosolids application to agricultural land began in the 1970s and was, and the EPA promoted it as a cost-effective soil amendment.

Large and small farms adopted this practice to improve soil and crop yields. However, many farmers remain unaware of PFAS contamination in biosolids, which leads to PFAS accumulation in crops and livestock. Contaminated farms face economic losses and health risks. The Environmental Working Group estimates that 20 million acres of US farmland contain contamination. This widespread issue affects food production and rural communities.

PFAS contamination occurs in thousands of locations across the USA and worldwide. Maine identifies 59 PFAS-contaminated farms through soil and water testing by state environmental agencies. Other states lag in testing, leaving the full extent unknown. Experts predict hundreds more farms will discover contamination soon.

PFAS uptake varies among crops, with leafy greens and root vegetables absorbing more than grains. Grocery stores and farmers' markets do not label produce's PFAS content. Livestock living on contaminated properties consume PFAS. Consumers unknowingly purchase contaminated beef, pork, poultry, milk, cream, ice cream, and butter.

Maine farmers euthanize hundreds of cows due to high PFAS levels. A New Mexico dairy culls 4,000 cows after milk tests positive for PFAS. The Tozier farm in Maine stops selling milk and beef, losing its primary income. Fred Stone's multi-generational dairy farm shuts down, killing contaminated livestock. Farmers face lost revenue, decreased property values, and costs for water filtration. Maine establishes a $60 million fund to assist impacted farmers. This crisis affects agricultural communities nationwide. The lack of widespread testing and labeling leaves consumers vulnerable to PFAS exposure through food.

Farmers need support to transition away from using contaminated biosolids. Maine established a $60 million fund to assist impacted farmers. The program provides income replacement, water filtration, and land buyouts at pre-contamination value. Massachusetts developed a similar relief fund. Most states lack support programs, leaving farmers to bear the costs alone. Contaminated farmland faces uncertain futures.

Some farmers switch to crops that are less prone to PFAS uptake, while others install water filtration systems to continue operations. Contaminated land may remain fallow for decades. Maine is considering purchasing affected farms for long-term management. Solar development emerges as an alternative use for contaminated fields. Research explores remediation options for PFAS-tainted soil. The Aroostook Band of Micmacs in Maine uses hemp to extract PFAS from soil.

This phytoremediation shows promise but requires proper disposal of contaminated plants. Scientists investigate other plant species and soil treatments to remove PFAS. Complete cleanup of contaminated farmland may take generations. The USDA offers assistance for PFAS testing through the Environmental Quality Incentives Program. EPA awards $15 million for research on PFAS exposure and reduction in agriculture.

Collaborative efforts between scientists, policymakers, and farmers pave the way for safer agricultural practices. Innovative solutions and public awareness remain crucial to break the cycle of PFAS contamination.

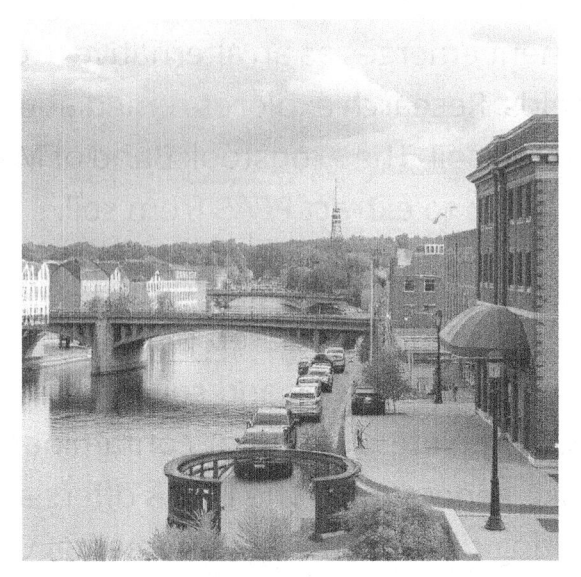

Chapter 6

The PFAS Nightmare: DuPont in Parkersburg

In 1951, DuPont began using PFOA to manufacture Teflon at its Washington Works plant near Parkersburg, West Virginia. This decision marked the beginning of a decades-long environmental disaster. By 1961, DuPont learned it was toxic but continued using it, keeping this information hidden from the public. In 1979, a DuPont survey found evidence of liver damage in Teflon plant employees, raising internal concerns. These early warning signs went unheeded as production continued.

The 1980s bring more evidence of PFOA's dangers. In 1981, 3M and DuPont reassigned female workers after animal studies revealed that PFAS damages fetal eyes. This demonstrates early knowledge of reproductive risks. By 1984, DuPont detected PFAS in tap water in Little Hocking, Ohio, but didn't alert the local water utility. This begins a pattern of concealment that will last for years.

In the 1990s, DuPont's contamination escalated. From 1990 to 1996, the company dumped 7,100 tons of PFOA-laced sludge into unlined "digestion ponds" on the Washington Works property. They also created the Dry Run Landfill for hazardous PFOA disposal. In 1993, West Virginia Department of Environmental Protection inspectors found "excessive amounts of sediment and discoloration" in the Dry Run Landfill property ponds. DuPont responded by draining contaminated leachate into Dry Run Creek.

The consequences of DuPont's actions became apparent in October 1996. Wilbur Earl Tennant, a farmer near Parkersburg, noticed his cows becoming sick and dying. Dry Run Creek, which runs through his 700-acre farm, turned black, foamed up, and smelled foul. This marked the beginning of public awareness of the contamination. In 1997, a DuPont study found heightened cancer rates among Parkersburg plant workers, further showing health risks.

The legal battle began in 1998 when Tennant hired lawyer Robert Bilott to investigate the cause of his cattle's deaths. In 1999, Bilott discovered DuPont's internal documents revealing massive PFOA emissions from the Washington Works plant. These documents show 24,000 pounds of annual air and 55,000 pounds of water emissions. This discovery sets the stage for a protracted legal fight.

The new millennium saw the first legal actions against DuPont. In 2000, Bilott filed a lawsuit against DuPont on behalf of Tennant, which settled for an undisclosed amount. In 2001, Bilott filed a class action lawsuit representing 70,000 people in six water districts near Parkersburg: Lubeck, Little Hocking, Belpre, Tuppers Plains, Mason County, and Pomeroy. The lawsuit brought national attention to the issue.

In 2004, the EPA sued DuPont for failing to report PFOA risks. Tests showed that Parkersburg residents had PFOA levels up to 128 ppb, far above the U.S. average of 5 ppb. This revelation shocked the community and intensified the legal battle. In 2005, DuPont settled with the EPA for $16.5 million, agreeing to remediate drinking water with PFOA levels exceeding 0.4 ppb. The EPA uses this money for PFOA research and to fund residents' blood tests.

The late 2000s and early 2010s brought increased scrutiny and regulation. In 2009, the EPA established a provisional health advisory level for PFOA at 0.4 ppb in drinking water. In 2012, the C8 Science Panel, funded by the class action settlement, found probable links between PFOA exposure and six diseases. These diseases include kidney cancer, testicular cancer, ulcerative colitis, thyroid disease, pregnancy-induced hypertension, and high cholesterol. This scientific evidence strengthens the case against DuPont.

In 2015, DuPont attempted to shield itself from liability by spinning off its Teflon division into Chemours. This move was criticized as an attempt to protect assets from legal claims. In 2016, the EPA lowered its health advisory level for PFOA to 0.07 ppb, reflecting growing concerns about the chemical's toxicity. These actions increased pressure on DuPont to address the contamination.

The legal consequences for DuPont began to mount in 2017. DuPont and Chemours paid $670.7 million to settle 3,550 personal injury lawsuits. The money was divided among the plaintiffs based on disease type and severity. This settlement marks a huge victory for the affected communities. In 2019, the film Dark Waters dramatized the story, increasing public awareness of the PFAS contamination issue.

The 2020s bring further settlements and attempts at remediation. In 2023, Ohio secured a $110 million settlement with DuPont for environmental restoration along the Ohio River. The funds will be used for water quality monitoring, habitat restoration, and public education programs. In 2024, a federal judge approved a $1.19 billion settlement for water contamination claims against DuPont and related companies.

This brings the total payout to over $2 billion. The Parkersburg PFAS contamination saga reveals a decades-long struggle for justice. DuPont repeatedly concealed information and contaminated the local environment, prioritizing profits over public health. The total payout represents less than the full scope of the long-term impact on the community.

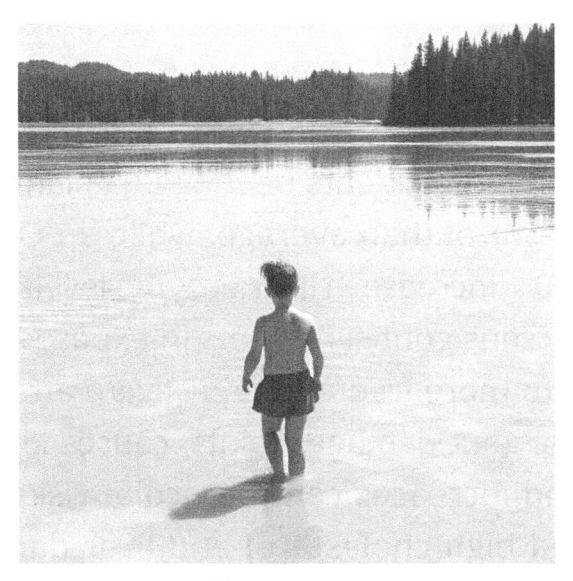

Chapter 7

PFAS and Human Health

PFAS enter human bodies through water, food, and consumer products, affecting 97% of the global population. Contaminated drinking water is the primary exposure route, with 95% of U.S. water sources and 80% of global supplies containing PFAS. Levels vary, but areas near industrial plants, manufacturing sites, and waste dumps often show significantly higher concentrations. For example, water near a fluorochemical plant in

West Virginia had PFOA levels of 3,500 parts per trillion (ppt), far exceeding the EPA's advisory limit of 70 ppt.

Short-term health effects include elevated cholesterol, liver enzymes, and uric acid levels. A 2018 North Carolina study found residents near a PFAS plant had 30% higher cholesterol than average, while an Ohio study revealed a 50% increase in liver enzyme levels. Elevated uric acid worsens gout symptoms in exposed individuals, leading to more frequent and severe attacks. Over time, chronic gout damages joints, causes kidney dysfunction, and increases cardiovascular risks. Similarly, untreated high cholesterol and liver damage can progress into fatty liver disease, inflammation, fibrosis, or cirrhosis.

PFAS also weakens the immune system, increasing susceptibility to infections and worsening illnesses. A 2013 Faroe Islands study showed children with high PFAS exposure had a 25% reduction in vaccine antibody production. During the COVID-19 pandemic, individuals with high PFAS levels experienced more severe symptoms and higher mortality rates. In Italy, deaths were 60% higher in a PFAS-contaminated region compared to less affected areas. Reduced efficacy of vaccines and medications in exposed populations further complicates treatment outcomes. For example, a Swedish study found that flu vaccines were 20% less effective in people with elevated PFAS levels.

Long-term health impacts include kidney cancer, thyroid disease, decreased vaccine response, ulcerative colitis, and pregnancy-induced hypertension. In the U.S., an estimated 200,000 people have PFAS-related kidney cancer; globally, this figure reaches 2 million. Children exposed to PFAS face developmental delays and reduced birth weight affecting about 15% of exposed infants. This can lead to lifelong complications such as delayed growth or chronic health issues. Moreover, delayed puberty onset in girls raises their risk of breast cancer later in life.

PFAS contamination has persisted for decades due to their resistance to degradation. These chemicals accumulate in the blood, liver, and kidneys and remain in the body for years, with half-lives ranging from three to eight years. Despite their widespread presence and health risks, public awareness has lagged behind exposure levels.

PFAS bioaccumulate in the blood, liver, kidneys, and other tissues because they resist breakdown in the human body. This process was first documented in the 1970s through occupational exposure studies, such as those conducted on workers at a fluorochemical plant in West Virginia. PFAS enters the bloodstream through ingestion, inhalation, or skin contact and binds to proteins, allowing them to circulate and deposit in organs. PFAS disrupts fat metabolism in the liver, increasing fatty liver disease risk. The kidneys impair filtration and excretion processes, potentially causing nephrotoxicity and kidney stones. These chemicals persist for years, with half-lives ranging from 3 to 8 years.

Unlike lead poisoning, no definitive body burden threshold has been established for PFAS exposure. However, higher PFAS levels correlate with increased health risks. Continuous exposure compounds existing conditions such as high cholesterol, liver damage, and hyperuricemia. For example, individuals with gout who have elevated PFAS levels experience more frequent and severe attacks. Chronic gout can lead to joint deformities, kidney disease, and cardiovascular complications. Similarly, elevated cholesterol from PFAS exposure increases fatty deposits in arteries, raising heart disease risks. Persistent liver damage may progress to fibrosis or cirrhosis over time.

PFAS disrupts the endocrine system, which regulates hormones critical for growth, metabolism, and reproduction. This disruption contributes to metabolic disorders like obesity and diabetes by altering glucose regulation and fat storage. In the U.S., obesity affects over

40% of adults, diabetes impacts 11%, and cardiovascular diseases remain the leading cause of death. Globally, obesity rates exceed 13%, with diabetes affecting 10% of adults. Ironically, while people avoid fatty foods like chips to lower cholesterol, they may unknowingly consume PFAS-contaminated smoothies made with polluted fruit in plastic containers.

Exposure also reduces bone density by interfering with calcium metabolism, increasing osteoporosis risk. In the U.S., 10 million people have osteoporosis; worldwide, this figure rises to over 200 million. Hormonal disruption from PFAS affects reproductive health by altering estrogen and testosterone levels. This can harm fetal development and increase mental health issues such as depression and anxiety due to imbalanced hormone r egulation.PFAS weakens immune function by suppressing antibody production and reducing vaccine efficacy.

Studies show that 97% of Americans have detectable PFAS in their blood, but only 7% have detailed levels measured through programs like National Health and Nutrition Examination Survey know as NHANES. This discrepancy arises because NHANES focuses on specific PFAS compounds and uses blood tests as a proxy for exposure. PFAS contamination spans every continent globally, with hotspots near manufacturing sites, military bases, and industrial areas. For example, in the

U.S., water near fluorochemical plants often exceeds EPA safety limits.

Specific populations face disproportionate exposure risks. Communities near industrial facilities or military bases often experience contamination levels far above regulatory thresholds. For example, 31% of groundwater samples near known PFAS sources in the U.S. exceed EPA limits, compared to 6% in areas without direct sources. Occupational exposure is also significant; firefighters, chemical plant workers, and ski wax technicians have higher PFAS levels due to contact with contaminated materials. Studies show these groups experience elevated risks of cancer, liver disease, and immune dysfunction. For instance, firefighters exposed to PFAS foam report 20-30% higher cancer rates than the general population.

Socioeconomic factors also influence exposure. Disadvantaged communities often live closer to contaminated sites or rely on polluted water sources due to limited resources. Indigenous populations relying on traditional foods like fish or game usually face higher PFAS exposure because these foods bioaccumulate chemicals from contaminated ecosystems. For example, studies in Alaska show elevated PFAS levels in subsistence fishers consuming local salmon.

PFAS exposure compounds health issues across generations due to its persistence and bioaccumulation. It disrupts metabolic processes and the endocrine system, which regulates hormones critical for growth and reproduction. This disruption increases risks for obesity, diabetes, and cardiovascular disease by altering fat storage and glucose regulation.

Prenatal and early childhood exposure to PFAS raises large health concerns. PFAS crosses the placental barrier, transferring from mother to fetus through blood circulation. This process disrupts fetal growth by interfering with the placenta's nutrient transport, hormone secretion, and waste removal. Studies in North Carolina and Japan link higher PFAS levels to reduced birth weight, preterm delivery, and gestational hypertension. For example, a U.S. study found a 29-gram reduction in fetal weight per unit increase in PFOS exposure.

Breastfeeding transfers PFAS from mother to infant as these chemicals bind to proteins in breast milk. Ironically, mothers often breastfeed believing it is healthier, unaware their milk may contain higher PFAS levels than formula unless it is stored in plastic containers. Children face heightened exposure risks because they consume more food and water relative to body weight than adults. This increased intake magnifies PFAS accumulation during critical developmental stages.

PFAS exposure during early life affects growth, cognition, and immune function. Disruption of thyroid hormones impairs brain development, increasing the risks for neurodevelopmental disorders like autism spectrum disorder (ASD) and developmental delays (DD). A California study found that elevated PFAS levels in children aged 2-5 correlated with higher ASD and DD diagnoses. As PFAS interferes with metabolic pathways essential for tissue development, growth deficits also occur.

Immune function suffers as PFAS suppresses antibody production and weakens vaccine responses. Children exposed to high PFAS levels show reduced infection resistance and slower recovery times. Cognitive impacts include lower IQ scores and impaired memory due to disrupted neurochemical signaling during brain development.

The long-term effects of early PFAS exposure compound over time. These include increased risks of obesity, diabetes, cardiovascular disease, and osteoporosis later in life. For instance, metabolic disruption caused by PFAS alters fat storage and glucose regulation, contributing to the 40% obesity rate in U.S. adults. Hormonal imbalances also affect mental health, increasing risks for anxiety and depression due to disrupted estrogen and testosterone levels.

PFAS exposure poses significant risks to human health across all stages of life, from prenatal development to adulthood. Its persistence in the body and environment ensures that its effects compound over time, creating long-term health obstacles for individuals and communities. Despite growing awareness of these dangers, much remains unknown about the full extent of PFAS's impact on human health.

The next chapter will explore how PFAS contamination affects wildlife. These chemicals, from aquatic ecosystems to land animals, disrupt natural habitats and threaten biodiversity worldwide.

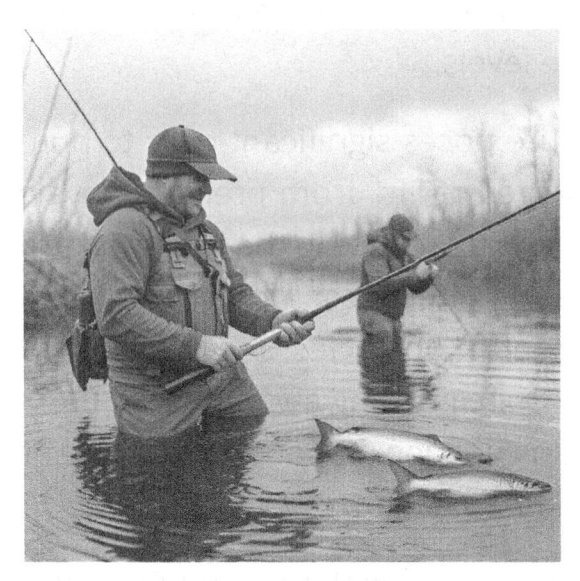

Chapter 8

Wildlife, Birds, Fish Fisherman and Hunters

P FAS contamination is a global menace, threatening wildlife and ecosystems on a massive scale. With over 600 species affected across continents, these "forever chemicals" seep into food chains via polluted water, soil, and air, inflicting irreversible health damage on numerous animals. From the Arctic to Florida's wetlands, no species is immune to the reach of PFAS.

In North Carolina's Cape Fear River, American alligators battle PFAS from the Chemours plant, which DuPont operated from 1971 to 2015. This contamination spans over 300 miles of waterways, with all tested alligators carrying PFAS in their blood. Liver concentrations in these reptiles average 10 ppb, ten times higher than in cleaner habitats. The alligators exhibit unhealed lesions and autoimmune conditions, with interferon-alpha genes 400 times more active than usual. This mirrors human lupus patients, showing the parallels between wildlife and human health impacts.

The Arctic is in the grip of a PFAS crisis, with polar bears bearing the brunt of alarming contamination levels. A 2023 study unveiled average PFOS concentrations of 2.5 ppb in liver samples from over 50 bears. These chemicals, transported via atmospheric currents and ocean pathways, trigger thyroid dysfunction and reduce cub survival in polar bears. The situation mirrors thyroid issues seen in human populations near PFAS hotspots, underscoring the shared nature of this environmental threat.

Tigers in India's Sundarbans and Russia's Primorsky Krai are contaminated with PFAS from textile factories that discharge chemicals into nearby rivers. Blood serum tests of 12 tigers revealed PFOS levels averaging 1.2 ppb, leading to liver enlargement and reduced hunting efficiency. This contamination poses a significant threat to already endangered populations, emphasizing the urgent need to protect these vulnerable species from the compounding effects of PFAS.

In Thailand's Khao Yai National Park, long-tailed macaques show PFAS exposure through agricultural runoff. Fifteen monkeys tested in 2023 had PFOS levels of 0.8 ppb and PFOA levels of 0.45 ppb, leading to developmental delays and abnormal cortisol levels. Similarly, China's giant pandas in the Qinling Mountains suffer from PFAS contamination linked to electronics manufacturing. Fecal samples showed PFOS at 1.1 ppb, causing liver enzyme abnormalities and suppressed vaccine responses.

Marine mammals are not spared from the impacts of PFAS. Bottlenose dolphins in South Carolina's Charleston Harbor had PFAS levels averaging three ppb in their blood plasma. Biopsies revealed chronic inflammation and liver fibrosis, with calf mortality rates increasing by 30% post-exposure. The liver damage seen in these dolphins mirrors human liver disease linked to PFAS exposure, further emphasizing the interconnectedness of environmental and human health.

Migratory birds at Holloman Lake, New Mexico, face significant PFAS exposure from US Air Force firefighting foam used since the 1970s. Mallards averaged 12.4 ppb PFOS in their livers, while killdeer reached 32 ppb. Over 100 migratory bird species ingest PFAS through contaminated invertebrates and rodents, leading to nest failures and unhatched eggs.

The impact extends beyond wildlife to livestock, posing risks to food safety and agricultural economies. In Clovis, New Mexico, 3,665 cows were euthanized after milk tested at six ppb PFOS, far exceeding the FDA limit of 0.02 ppb. This contamination, stemming from Cannon Air Force Base, resulted in $5.9 million in losses for Highland Dairy. The incident shows the economic devastation PFAS can wreak on farming communities.

PFAS contamination in livestock is a global concern. While 550 chicken samples tested by the USDA showed no PFAS detections, studies in China found PFOS (25.7 ppb) and PFOA (4.75 ppb) in chicken livers near industrial zones. Pigs show widespread contamination, with 100% of pigs tested at a Swedish farm linked to contaminated feed showing PFAS presence. In China, pig livers contained PFOS (4.29 ppb) from industrial wastewater used for irrigation.

Aquatic ecosystems face severe PFAS impacts. Holloman Lake invertebrates contain 1.1-77 ppb PFAS, transferred to predators like ducks and fish. Cape Fear River plankton also shows PFAS contamination, affecting the base of marine food webs. These contaminated invertebrates serve as vectors, moving PFAS up the food chain and potentially into human diets.

PFAS contamination in game fish poses serious health risks, with measurements expressed in nanograms per kilogram (ng/kg)—1 ng equals one-billionth of a gram. The EPA's health advisory for PFOS in water is 0.02 ng/L, roughly equivalent to 1,000 ng/kg in fish tissue. Fish with PFAS levels exceeding 1,000 ng/kg are considered unsafe, as consuming them is comparable to drinking 290 times the EPA's monthly limit for water. Minnesota's guidelines treat PFOS in fish even more strictly, considering it 10 times more dangerous than mercury or PCBs.

Trout and bass, popular game fish, are contaminated at alarming levels across the United States. Rainbow trout from federal hatcheries in the Northeast have PCB levels so high that consumption should be limited to one meal every two months or less. Largemouth bass average between 9,397 and 41,219 ng/kg PFAS nationally, while trout in Lake Seneca, New York, contain 11,800 to 44,000 ng/kg PFOS. Smallmouth bass in US rivers have been found with up to 28,227 ng/kg PFAS.

Despite these health risks and advisories, many fishermen and sportsmen consume contaminated fish. This behavior stems from a combination of tradition, lack of awareness, and the cultural significance of fishing. The conflict between health warnings and deeply ingrained practices poses issues for public health officials and environmental agencies. The impact of fish contamination extends beyond individual health risks. Sportfishing economies face potential losses due to fishing advisories and reduced fish consumption. However, many anglers prioritize their cultural practices and traditions over health warnings, creating a complex situation for environmental management and public health initiatives.

PFAS contamination plagues major U.S. waterways, and several emerging hotspots show extreme pollution levels. The Cape Fear River in North Carolina is heavily polluted, with fish PFOS levels reaching 1,364.7 ppt (83 times the EPA limit) due to Chemours/DuPont operations from 1971 to 2015. Nearby, GenX contamination in water reaches 25.8 ppt from Fayetteville manufacturing. In Maryland, Piscataway Creek near Washington D.C. shows PFOS levels of 1,364.7 ppt in water, a staggering 68,235 times the EPA advisory level.

Pennsylvania's Kreutz Creek suffers from industrial runoff, with PFOA levels in the water at 847 ppt, 211,750 times the EPA limit. The Conasauga River in Georgia exhibits the state's highest PFAS levels downstream of

Dalton's carpet factories. New York's Niagara River contains over 35 PFAS compounds near industrial zones. Green Bay's groundwater in Wisconsin shows alarming PFOS concentrations of 1.9 million ppt, attributed to Air Force firefighting foam use.

The Chattahoochee River in Georgia has triggered EPA warnings due to PFAS contamination in bass near Atlanta. Lake Superior faces a multi-state advisory as rainbow smelt shows PFOS levels of 280,000 ppt. The Savannah River, straddling Georgia and South Carolina, deals with this pollution, including toxaphene and PFAS from textile and chemical plants. Even the Great Lakes basin isn't spared, with rain depositing 10-70 ppt of atmospheric PFAS across all five lakes.

Specific fish species show concerning contamination levels. Largemouth bass in the Cape Fear River contain up to 41,219 ng/kg PFAS. Rainbow trout in Lake Seneca, NY, reach 44,000 ng/kg PFOS. Channel catfish in Illinois' Rock River average 9,500 ng/kg PFAS. These levels pose significant risks to consumers, with health experts warning that eating one Great Lakes fish is equivalent to drinking PFAS-tainted water for a month.

Primary pollution sources include over 100 military bases with PFAS levels exceeding 100,000 ppt, textile mills in Dalton, GA, discharging into the Conasauga River, and electronics manufacturing, contributing to high PFAS loads in Pennsylvania waterways. The widespread nature of this contamination shows the urgent need for comprehensive remediation efforts and stricter regulations on PFAS use across industries.

It's not just fishermen who consume poisoned fish—hunters risk ingesting PFAS, lead, and industrial toxins through deer, wild boar, rabbits, upland birds, and waterfowl. These chemicals persist in animals that migrate between contaminated and clean areas, creating invisible health risks.

Deer have become silent carriers of PFAS in several regions. In Maine, "Do Not Eat" advisories cover 34 square miles in Fairfield, Unity, and Albion after deer tested at 547 ppb PFOS. These contaminated fields, caused by sludge since the 1970s, have poisoned browsing herds. Michigan's Clark's Marsh deer average 250 ppb PFAS in liver, with one individual hitting 547 ppb in muscle. Alarmingly, migrating deer can spread toxins more than 15 miles from the origin sites. Health experts warn that consuming eight or more meals per year from tainted zones risks liver damage and thyroid dysfunction.

Wild boars in Europe have become mobile toxic reservoirs. In the Bohemian Forest of Czechia, boar livers average 230 μg/kg PFAS, five times the EU limits, with industrial PFOS/PFOA being dominant. Northeastern Germany's rural boars carry 110 μg/kg PFAS from atmospheric deposition. The consumption risk is significant—eating just 100g of liver annually exceeds EU toxicity thresholds for cancer and fertility harm.

Small game and upland birds are not spared from contamination. At Holloman Lake in New Mexico, kangaroo rats hit 120,000 ppb PFAS, and rabbits grazing on contaminated vegetation likely absorb similar levels. Iowa cottontails near industrial zones show lead fragments from ammunition—ruffed grouse near PFAS-treated crops in Iowa average eight ppb PFOS in muscle. Globally, lead poisoning from shot affects 30% of hunter-harvested birds.

Waterfowl act as migratory PFAS vectors. American wigeon at Holloman Lake reach 38,000 ppb PFAS, where consuming just 1g of meat exceeds EPA lifetime limits. In Victoria, Australia, ducks carry 12 ppb PFOS from textile runoff. Black ducks in the Northeast US average 9,397 ng/kg PFAS, prompting advisories limiting consumption to two meals per month.

The nomadic nature of these animals exacerbates the spread of contamination. Deer can travel over 20 miles, transferring PFAS from industrial zones to clean forests. Migratory birds, like ducks at Holloman Lake, carry PFAS to Canada's wetlands within weeks. Wild boar's rooting behavior spreads soil-bound PFAS across more than 10 square miles annually.

Health agencies confirm that no safe cooking method removes PFAS from meat. Despite advisories, cultural practices drive consumption—67% of Maine hunters eat venison from restricted zones. This widespread contamination shows the urgent need for comprehensive remediation efforts, stricter regulations on PFAS use across industries, and increased public awareness about the risks of consuming game from affected areas.

Insects, significant to Earth's ecosystems, face unprecedented declines due to PFAS. Studies reveal PFAS bioaccumulation in aquatic insects like midges and dragonflies (1.1–77 ppb PFAS), which then transfer toxins to terrestrial predators. Agricultural runoff from PFAS-treated crops further poisons pollinators. Fruit flies exposed to 6 ppb PFOS showed a 60% reduction in egg-laying rates, illustrating the chemicals' impact on insect reproduction. The decline in insect populations threatens to collapse entire food webs, endangering 75% of food crops and starving fish, birds, and amphibians that rely on these insects for food.

The scale of PFAS contamination is staggering. Over 15,000 PFAS chemicals have been produced globally since the 1960s. A 2024 global study analyzed 45,000+ water samples, revealing that 31% of groundwater and 16% of surface water exceed safe PFAS levels. In the US alone, over 8,865 documented sites are contaminated, with 17,000+ sites in Europe and hotspots in Australia, China, and India. PFAS now taint millions of hectares of land, including 610 contaminated US locations and 53,000 tons of polluted soil in Germany's Rastatt region.

These chemicals persist for centuries, with PFOS and PFOA half-lives exceeding 1,000 years in soil and water. Even if production ceased today, existing PFAS would continue infiltrating ecosystems for generations. Studies show PFAS in rainwater exceeds safety limits globally, contaminating 75% of US crops and 20% of EU drinking water sources.

The persistence of PFAS poses long-term risks to ecosystem health and human safety. New Mexico's 2025 advisory warns that consuming just one gram of duck meat from Holloman Lake could exceed EPA's lifetime PFAS exposure limits. PFAS levels in the lake's water range from 5.9 to 16 ppt, up to 1,600 times EPA's drinking water limit of 4 ppt for PFOA and PFOS. This widespread contamination shows the urgent need for comprehensive remediation efforts and stricter regulations on PFAS use.

The chemicals persist in ecosystems, altering wildlife gene expression and threatening species' survival across global migratory routes. With 69% of global groundwater surpassing Canada's PFAS limits, humanity faces a toxic world that will impact planetary health for millennia.

The PFAS crisis demands immediate action to protect wildlife, ecosystems, and human health. Stricter regulations on PFAS production and use, improved water treatment technologies, and extensive cleanup efforts are needed.

Public awareness and engagement drive policy changes and market shifts from PFAS-containing products. The fate of countless species and the health of future generations depend on our collective response to this pervasive environmental threat.

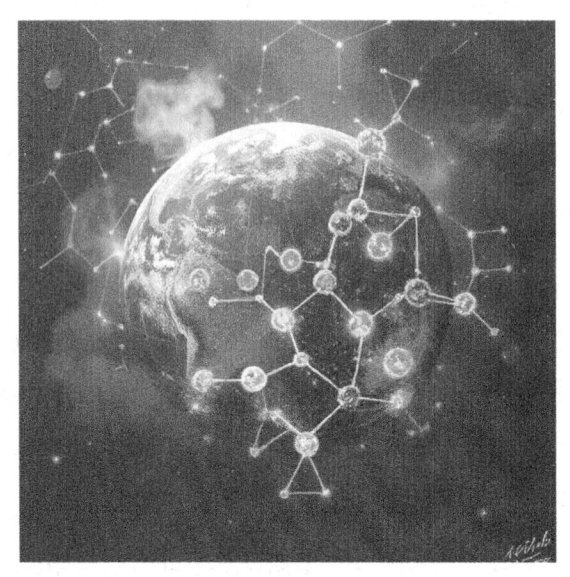

Chapter 9

Regulations

Due to their environmental persistence and potential health risks, the regulation of per- and poly-fluoroalkyl substances (PFAS) has become a global priority. In recent years, governments worldwide have implemented stricter regulations to mitigate chemical impact. This comprehensive overview examines the evolving regulatory criteria, focusing on recent regional bans and restrictions.

On April 10, 2024, the U.S. Environmental Protection Agency (EPA) finalized national primary drinking water regulations for six chemical compounds. The new rule establishes legally enforceable Maximum Contaminant Levels (MCLs) levels for PFOA, PFOS, PFHxS, PFNA, HFPO-DA, and chemical mixtures. Public water systems must monitor for these PFAS by 2027 and comply with standards by 2029.

The EPA estimates that 4,100 to 6,700 water systems, serving between 83 million and 105 million people, will need to reduce regulated forever chemicals. The regulation is expected to cost $1.63 billion per year, totaling more than $128 billion over 82 years. This cost includes the expenses for monitoring, treatment, and compliance. Water agencies have commented that the EPA's cost estimates are lower than their projections.

The EPA announced that $1 billion in funding is available through the Infrastructure Investment and Jobs Act to support implementation. This funding helps states and territories implement contaminant testing and treatment at public water systems and assists private property owners in addressing PFAS contamination.

On April 19, 2024, the EPA finalized a rule designating PFOA and PFOS, including their salts and structural isomers, as "hazardous substances" under Comprehensive Environmental Response, Compensation, and Liability Act, also known as Superfund and CERCLA. Effective July 8, 2024, this rule expands liability under the law and brings new obligations for the regulated community.

The EPA issued a "PFAS Enforcement Discretion and Settlement Policy Under CERCLA" on April 19, 2024. This policy provides a framework for holding responsible entities that have" contributed" to PFAS release, including manufacturers and industrial parties. It aims to strike a balance between enforcement and providing comfort for municipal entities and farmers applying biosolids to land, by allowing for discretion in certain cases.

In February 2023, the European Union proposed a comprehensive ban on non-essential PFAS uses. The EU adopted a phased approach to implementing PFAS regulations, with a 10-year transition period for critical applications like firefighting foams in offshore oil and gas operations. The EU emphasizes enforcement, with regulatory bodies like the European Chemicals Agency (ECHA) empowered to monitor compliance and impose penalties. The EU sets strict guidelines and penalties to ensure companies adhere to regulations.

Australia introduced regulatory measures focused on PFOA and related compounds. The Australian Industrial Chemicals Introduction Scheme (AICIS) requires importers and exporters to obtain authorization for PFOA-related compounds. This process involves submitting detailed information about the compound, its intended use, and its potential environmental and health impacts. Australia's approach aligns with the EU and U.S. international standards.

In the United States, the regulatory guidelines for these chemicals are more fragmented, with federal and state-level actions. The EPA proposes rules to prevent 300 PFAS chemicals from re-entering commerce. Companies must complete EPA reviews and risk assessments before manufacturing or processing certain "inactive PFAS" chemicals.

States have taken the initiative to implement stricter regulations. Minnesota bans the intentional use of PFAS in various consumer products starting January 1, 2025; manufacturers must report PFAS usage by January 1, 2026. Other states, like California and New York, have introduced laws to reduce foreign chemicals in food packaging and water supplies.

The global regulatory criteria for PFAS are evolving, and several key trends are emerging. There is a growing trend toward comprehensive bans over partial restrictions. Regulators are adopting phased implementation strategies to allow industries time to adjust and find safer alternatives.

Due to the critical nature of PFAS applications, specific industries, such as firefighting, may receive needed consideration. These sectors may get extended transition periods or allowances for continued use of certain PFAS compounds. Global coordination is improving as regulators in different countries collaborate on PFAS risk assessments and regulatory measures, providing reassurance about the collective effort in addressing this issue.

As concerns about PFAS contamination grow, regulatory bodies are adopting stronger enforcement mechanisms, including stricter penalties for non-compliance. This trend is observed across different regions, reflecting the increasing urgency to address PFAS-related issues and the gravity of the situation.

The designation of PFOA and PFOS as hazardous substances under CERCLA expands liability under the law. Responsible parties (PRPs) include current and past owners and operators of impacted property, generators, and hazardous waste transporters. A recent court decision reaffirms that knowledge is not a factor in the liability scheme.

The EPA's enforcement policy for forever chemicals under CERCLA focuses on parties contributing to PFAS release. Implementing this policy may prove difficult at sediment sites where most PFAS likely come from municipal discharges.

In the United Kingdom, the Health and Safety Executive (HSE) publishes a report on regulatory management options for PFAS. This report is the first step toward a UK PFAS restriction proposal that is expected to align with the EU proposal.

The Department of Defense (DoD) in the United States administers actions specific to defense personnel, operations, installations, and their immediate surroundings. In Canada, regulations are overseen by Environment and Climate Change Canada (ECCC) and its provincial offices. Mexico's Ministry of Environment has not yet regulated PFAS.

The Stockholm Convention on Persistent Organic Pollutants plays a significant role in shaping global PFAS regulations. It provides a framework for eliminating or reducing the production and use of persistent organic pollutants, including certain PFAS compounds.

The EPA's PFAS Strategic Roadmap, updated in November 2024, outlines the agency's comprehensive approach to addressing PFAS contamination. This strategy includes actions across various EPA programs, focusing on research, restriction, and remediation of PFAS. The National Defense Authorization Act (NDAA) has included increasing PFAS-related requirements since 2018.

The 2018 NDAA mandated a study on PFAS exposure and health implications in communities near military bases with known PFAS contamination. This comprehensive approach should instill confidence in the agency's commitment to addressing PFAS contamination. The funding for PFAS remediation and research comes from various sources. The EPA makes funding available through programs like the Infrastructure Investment and Jobs Act. States may allocate funds for PFAS-related initiatives. In some cases, responsible parties may be required to pay for cleanup and remediation efforts.

Enforcement of PFAS regulations varies by jurisdiction. In the U.S., the EPA and state environmental agencies are responsible for the needed enforcement. Member states and EU-level bodies like ECHA play key roles in ensuring compliance with PFAS regulations in the EU.

The costs associated with PFAS regulation and remediation are significant.

Water utilities, manufacturers, and other affected industries may bear substantial costs to comply with new standards. These costs may be passed on to consumers through increased prices for goods and services. The PFAS regulations continue to evolve and industries are adapting to new requirements. This includes developing alternative substances, modifying production processes, and implementing new treatment technologies.

The regulatory framework is expected to remain dynamic as scientific understanding of PFAS impacts grows. Global efforts to address PFAS contamination face obstacles due to these substances' ubiquity and persistence in the environment. Ongoing research aims to understand better PFAS behavior, health impacts, and effective remediation techniques. This research informs future regulatory decisions and policy approaches. The impact of PFAS regulations extends beyond environmental concerns.

Economic considerations, public health implications, and technological obstacles all shape policy decisions. Balancing these factors remains a key challenge for regulators and policymakers worldwide.

As PFAS regulations become more stringent, a growing focus is on developing and implementing effective remediation technologies. This includes advanced water treatment methods, soil remediation techniques, and strategies for addressing PFAS in various environmental media.\

The global nature of PFAS contamination necessitates international cooperation. Efforts to harmonize regulations, share scientific data, and coordinate enforcement actions are ongoing. Differences in regulatory approaches between countries and regions persist, creating difficulties for global industries.

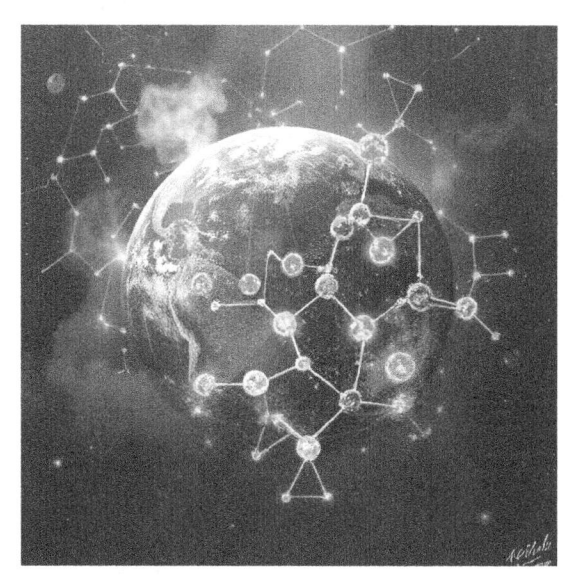

Chapter 10

PFAS Litigation

PFAS litigation has transcended borders, becoming a global phenomenon that unites legal professionals, environmental activists, policymakers, and industry stakeholders worldwide. This comprehensive overview jumps into the evolving legal framework, with a focus on recent lawsuits, settlements, and international developments. The sheer scale of the issue is evident in the fact that 3M is currently facing over 2,000 lawsuits related to PFAS contamination, with significant financial implications.

In 2021, DuPont and Chemours agreed to a $4 billion settlement, setting a precedent for future cases. These lawsuits allege that companies were aware of PFAS risks but continued production, often resulting in confidentiality agreements and limited public disclosure.

The financial implications of settlements are staggering. In 2024, 3M finalized a $12 billion settlement with public water systems for PFAS remediation, with payments spanning from 2024 to 2036. This settlement, one of the largest in PFAS legal action history, shows the financial burden on corporations and the long-term commitment required for remediation.

Tyco Fire Products agreed to a $750 million settlement in April 2024 for water contamination from firefighting foam. BASF settled for $316 million in May 2024 with U.S. public water systems over PFAS contamination. Carrier Global and its subsidiary Kidde-Fenwal paid $730 million in October 2024 to resolve firefighting foam claims.

Class action suits represent communities affected by PFAS contamination, often resulting in huge settlements. The Hoosick Falls, New York case resulted in a $65 million settlement, while Parkersburg, West Virginia residents received $671 million from DuPont.

Ongoing class actions include firefighters exposed to PFAS-containing foam and communities near contaminated sites. In November 2024, Nantucket residents filed a class action against DuPont, 3M, and BASF. Firefighter lawsuits have surged, with individual claims like the ulcerative colitis case in New York in October 2024.

Consumer product lawsuits are emerging as a new front in PFAS legal action. A class action against Kenvue and J&J in July 2024 alleges PFAS presence in Band-Aid products. Bic Razors faced similar claims in May 2024, expanding the scope of PFAS legal action beyond industrial contamination. State attorneys general are filing lawsuits against PFAS manufacturers to recover cleanup costs. In 2018, Minnesota settled with 3M for $850 million. New Jersey sued DuPont, Chemours, and 3M for environmental damage, seeking to shift remediation costs from taxpayers to polluters.

Recent state-level actions include the Texas Attorney General's lawsuit in December 2024 against PFAS manufacturers for deceptive practices.

Maryland expanded claims against Carrier Fire Americas and others in November 2024. Illinois and Alabama filed new PFAS lawsuits targeting 3M, Daikin, and Toray in 2024. The EPA's designation of PFOA and PFOS as "hazardous substances" under CERCLA in April 2024 has triggered Superfund liability. Superfund liability refers to the responsibility of potentially responsible parties (PRPs) to clean up hazardous waste sites. This regulatory change is expected to influence future litigation and corporate responsibility. State bans, such as Minnesota's 2025 PFAS ban on consumer products, also shape the legal framework.

PFAS contamination is a global issue showing the need for international cooperation in addressing this issue. This has led to international legal action. Australia faces class actions over firefighting foam contamination near military bases. The country has banned PFAS in firefighting foams and introduced industrial chemical regulations, aligning with global trends.

The European Union proposed a comprehensive ban on non-essential PFAS uses in February 2023. This phased prohibition includes a 10-year transition for critical sectors. The UK's Health and Safety Executive is preparing a PFAS restriction proposal aligned with the

EU's approach. These international efforts give hope for a coordinated global solution to the PFAS issue.

In Asia, Japan introduced PFAS limits in drinking water in 2023. China, while lagging in regulation, faces contamination hotspots, according to 2024 studies. Canada regulates PFAS under federal environmental laws, with provinces like Quebec enforcing stricter standards. PFAS legal action is driving changes in industry practices. Companies are phasing out long-chain PFAS production due to legal and regulatory pressure. Some manufacturers are investing in alternative chemicals to replace PFAS. Due to mounting legal pressure, the outdoor gear industry is shifting away from PFAS-based water repellents.

3M announced plans to phase out PFAS production by 2025. The company faces billions in potential liabilities from PFAS lawsuits. DuPont spun off its PFAS business to Chemours, transferring some legal liabilities and leading to subsequent litigation between the two companies. Food packaging companies are exploring PFAS-free alternatives for grease-resistant products. These industry shifts reflect the far-reaching impact of PFAS legal action on product development and corporate strategy. The legal framework is reshaping entire sectors and driving innovation in chemical alternatives.

PFAS lawsuits can take years to resolve, with class actions often lasting 5-10 years. Individual cases, such as those involving farmers, may settle faster but require 2-3 years. Legal costs and time investment can be substantial for plaintiffs, creating barriers to justice for some affected parties. Proving the source and extent of contamination can be difficult in agricultural cases. Farmers face unique legal action obstacles , accumulating agricultural losses over the years and complicating damage calculations. Some farmers join class actions, while others pursue individual cases, leading to varied legal outcomes.

When companies cannot pay, bankruptcy may limit victim compensation. Chapter 11 bankruptcy allows companies to reorganize and limit liability payments. Kidde-Fenwal, a subsidiary of Carrier Global, used this strategy to manage liabilities from over 4,400 lawsuits. Victims of PFAS contamination often receive limited compensation after legal fees. Lawyers take 30-40% of settlement amounts in contingency fees. Individual payouts may be small relative to health impacts and property damage, leading to dissatisfaction among class members.

Long-term health monitoring programs, which address ongoing health concerns, are sometimes included in settlements. However, given the extent of harm, many affected individuals feel settlements are inadequate. The disparity between corporate payouts and individual compensation remains a contentious issue. Plaintiff strategies are evolving, shifting from environmental claims to consumer fraud.

"Greenwashing" lawsuits, such as those against REI and Bic, represent this new approach. These cases allege deceptive marketing practices related to PFAS containing products, where companies mislead consumers about the environmental benefits of their products.

Judicial issues are shaping the legal framework. The American Water Works Association v. EPA case in 2024 contests PFAS drinking water limits. Courts are rejecting 3M's "federal contractor defense" in cases in Illinois and Vermont, expanding corporate liability. The 'federal contractor defense' is a legal doctrine that shields government contractors from liability for products they produce under government contracts. Its rejection in these cases signifies a shift in the legal framework, increasing corporate liability. Insurance battles are emerging as a significant aspect of PFAS legal action.

Companies like BASF and Tyco are pursuing insurers to cover settlement costs. These cases show the financial strain on corporations and the potential for significant changes in how PFAS liabilities are handled in the insurance industry, which could have far-reaching implications for future litigation and corporate risk management.

As PFAS legal action continues to evolve, it exposes corporate knowledge of health risks and increases scrutiny of chemical regulation. The outcomes of these cases will likely influence future regulatory approaches and corporate practices regarding PFAS and other emerging contaminants. This could lead to more stringent regulations, increased corporate responsibility, and a shift towards safer chemical alternatives, benefiting public health and the environment.

The global nature of PFAS contamination necessitates international cooperation, yet differences in legal systems and regulations create hurdles for global PFAS accountability. As the legal framework evolves, it will continue to shape industry practices, regulatory policies, and public awareness of PFAS-related issues worldwide.

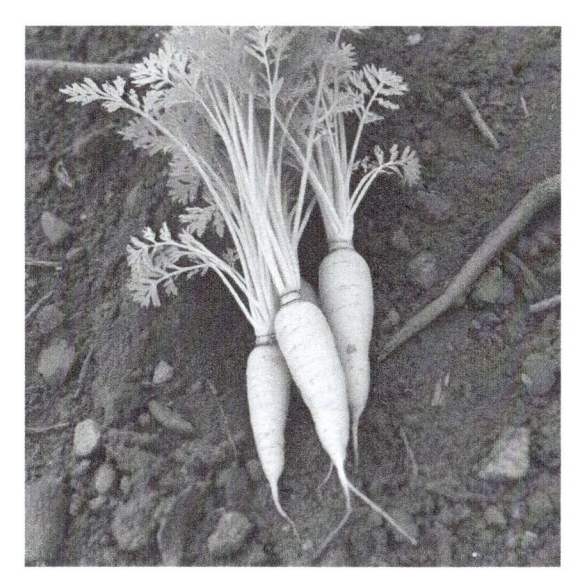

Chapter 11

PFAS in Fresh Produce

Farmers plant seeds in soil that hides this poison. As they grow, PFAS seeps into crops through roots, stems, and leaves. These chemicals bind to water molecules in the soil and hitchrides into plant tissues. Crops like lettuce and strawberries absorb them faster due to their shallow root systems. Even after harvest, residues cling to skins and leaves.

Pesticides like Fluroxypyr and Clopyralid, produced by Dow Chemical and BASF, contain PFAS as an inert ingredient. These formulas spread across fields, leaving chemical fingerprints on produce. Rainwater washes pesticide residues into the soil, creating long-term contamination reservoirs—PFAS-laced sludge fertilizers, approved for agriculture, further poison farmland. A single application taints soil for millennia.

Clay-rich soils trap PFAS, slowly releasing them to crops year after year. Sandy soils allow more profound chemical migration, contaminating groundwater and neighboring fields. Irrigation systems pump tainted water directly onto plants, accelerating uptake. Leafy greens like spinach absorb more PFAS through broad surface areas. Fruiting vegetables like tomatoes store chemicals in pulpy flesh.

Imported produce often carries higher risks due to lax regulations abroad. Mexican strawberries test with elevated PFAS levels from industrial wastewater irrigation. Chilean grapes show contamination from outdated pesticide use. Indian basmati rice plantations near textile factories absorb dye-related PFAS. Monitoring these imports remains inconsistent.

Strawberries are the most contaminated fruit, with 95% testing positive. Grapes follow at 61%, and peaches at 58%. Spinach leads vegetables at 42%, followed by tomatoes (38%) and cucumbers (34%). Nuts like almonds show lower but detectable levels of soil absorption.

Microwave popcorn bags and fast-food wrappers armor themselves with PFAS coatings. Brands like Orville Redenbacher use grease-resistant linings that leach chemicals when heated. Frozen pizza boxes from DiGiorno and Tombstone contain recycled fibers laced with PFAS. Canned soups from Campbell's and Progresso absorb toxins from epoxy resin linings—even "eco-friendly" compostable bowls at Chipotle harbor these chemicals.

PFAS invade boxed cereals through recycled cardboard packaging. General Mills Cheerios and Kellogg's Frosted Flakes show trace amounts in independent tests. Frozen meal trays from Lean Cuisine and Healthy Choice shed microplastics coated with PFAS. —Granola wrappers like Nature Valley's use water-resistant linings that degrade into food.

The microwave becomes a delivery system for contamination. Heating releases PFAS from popcorn bags into kernels. Steaming frozen vegetables in their plastic pouches transfers chemicals to food. Reheating takeout in containers accelerates chemical migration. Dishwasher-safe plastic meal kits accumulate PFAS through repeated heating cycles.

Cardboard food boxes made with recycled materials carry historical PFAS from past uses. Pizza Hut's delivery boxes contain fibers from old food wrappers and industrial papers. Cereal makers like Post blend virgin and recycled pulp, forever chemical toxins into new packaging. Soy-based inks on printed boxes do little to offset chemical risks

Our final discussion will confront life on a PFAS-saturated Earth. We must learn to navigate shrinking timelines for health and longevity. If we act swiftly, adaptation strategies may buy back precious years. The clock ticks louder now.

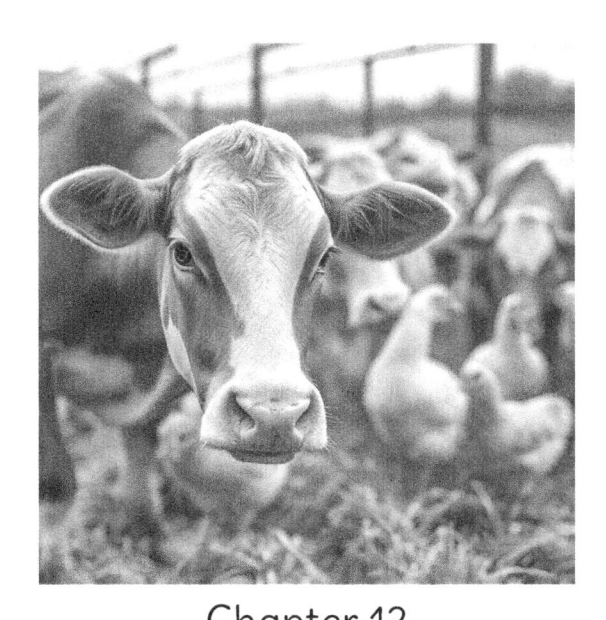

Chapter 12

So What Can We Do?

Y ou've reached the most crucial chapter - what to do about the PFAS contamination crisis. Our planet faces widespread pollution in water, food, and everyday items. With 97% of people harboring PFAS in their blood, the health risks are undeniable. We now confront a daunting reality: the invisibility of these harmful chemicals in our daily lives. Our food has no labels indicating PFAS content or exposure during production and packaging. This lack of transparency leaves us vulnerable and uninformed.

Tackling this issue requires a complete lifestyle overhaul. It's not a temporary diet or short-term project but a fundamental shift in how we interact with our environment. The goal is to minimize PFAS exposure to protect our health and extend our lives.

Let's start with everyday items. Say goodbye to disposable coffee cups and soft drinks in plastic bottles. Their unclear PFAS content makes them risky choices. At home, ditch plastic and paper plates for ceramic and glass alternatives. Yes, washing dishes takes effort, but it reduces PFAS exposure.

Opt for stainless steel, wood, or bamboo utensils and cooking tools. Avoid plastic kitchenware, as heat can cause it to leach chemicals. Invest in a stainless steel or glass thermos instead of plastic containers for on-the-go beverages.

Storage solutions need an overhaul, too. Replace plastic Tupperware with glass or ceramic containers. While some plastics claim to be safe, history teaches us to be skeptical. Remember the Parkersburg, Ohio tragedy where 70,000 people were poisoned for decades?

In the kitchen, use stainless steel, ceramic, or cast-iron cookware. Forget about nonstick pans, regardless of their convenience. Thorough washing is needed for food prep. Vinegar is an excellent multipurpose cleaning agent for produce and surfaces.

Maybe use a waterpik and wood toothpicks instead of dental floss. That might be a tough one.

Consider transforming your yard into a vegetable garden. Growing your produce with sourced soil in large containers helps control PFAS exposure. Opt for heirloom seeds and focus on plants native to your region. In Ohio, for example, berries thrive well.

Sourcing meat and poultry can be difficult. If possible, find organic or Amish producers. Otherwise, research your options and consider reducing the consumption of processed foods laden with preservatives and GMOs.

Your garden can do double duty by growing herbs for cooking and tea-making. Oregano, mint, parsley, and chamomile are easy to cultivate and can be used to make delicious PFAS-free beverages. Homemade herbal teas can replace store-bought soft drinks, saving money and reducing chemical exposure.

Expand your herb garden beyond the basics. Thyme, rosemary, and sage offer robust flavors for cooking.

Lemon balm, catnip, and hibiscus make refreshing iced teas. These plants thrive in raised beds or large pots, away from contaminated ground soil.

Create a dedicated tea garden with peppermint, spearmint, and lavender varieties. Dry excess herbs for year-round use. Experiment with blends to find your perfect caffeine-free pick-me-up. Herbal teas not only taste great but also offer various health benefits.

For soil, seek out leaf humus from uncontaminated forests or create your compost. Rotate crops annually to maintain soil health. Consider vertical gardening to maximize space and yield. With creativity, even small balconies can become productive herb havens.

Clothing choices matter, too. Favor natural fabrics like cotton, wool, and cashmere over synthetic materials. For footwear, leather or fabric options are preferable to plastic-based shoes. While we can't eliminate all synthetic materials, being mindful of our choices helps.

Home furnishings present another opportunity for reducing PFAS exposure. Consider natural fabric coverings for furniture and car seats. Avoid fabric softeners and opt for natural cleaning solutions for surfaces and laundry. YouTube offers many DIY cleaning product tutorials.

Create your all-purpose cleaner with vinegar, water, and essential oils. Baking soda works wonders on tough stains and odors. For laundry, try soap nuts or castile soap instead of conventional detergents. These alternatives are clean and without harsh chemicals.

Tackle shower cleaning with a mixture of hydrogen peroxide and water. Use microfiber cloths to reduce paper towel waste. Lemon juice cuts through soap scum naturally. For floors, a simple solution of hot water and a few drops of dish soap works wonders.

Water filtration is needed. Invest in a system that removes PFAS and other contaminants from your drinking and cooking water. If possible, extend filtration to shower and cleaning water. A whole-house purification system may be expensive but is considered a health investment.

Be mindful of environments with strong chemical odors, like new furniture stores. When vacationing, opt for ocean swimming over-chlorinated pools. Bring your drinks to the beach to avoid pool-side PFAS exposure.

Personal care products, too, require scrutiny. Many sunscreens, lotions, and cosmetics contain PFAS. Research PFAS-free alternatives and consider making your simple skincare products using natural ingredients. For example, you can make a natural sunscreen using zinc oxide, coconut oil, and shea butter. You can also create a moisturizing body butter with cocoa butter and essential oils. For hair care, try apple cider vinegar rinses and coconut oil masks. These DIY options reduce chemical exposure and save money.

Replace conventional deodorants with natural alternatives, such as crystal stones or homemade versions made with baking soda and arrowroot powder. Opt for mineral-based makeup and PFAS-free nail polishes. Every small change can reduce chemical exposure.

This lifestyle shift may be overwhelming but remember: it's about protecting yourself, not saving the entire planet single-handedly. By reducing your PFAS exposure, you're taking control of your health and extending your life.

Implementing these changes gradually can make the process more manageable. Start with one area, such as kitchen utensils or water filtration, and expand from there. Every small step reduces overall PFAS exposure and contributes to better health.

Education is key in this journey. Stay informed about new research and regulations regarding PFAS. Share your knowledge with friends and family to create a broader awareness of these issues. Collective action can lead to wider changes in product manufacturing and environmental policies.

Remember, while we can't eliminate PFAS exposure in our modern world, we can reduce it. This proactive approach empowers us to navigate a contaminated environment more safely, potentially mitigating long-term health risks.

As we conclude this exploration of PFAS contamination and mitigation strategies, let's embrace this knowledge as a tool for positive change. Your journey towards a lower-PFAS lifestyle starts now, armed with information and practical steps to create a healthier living environment.

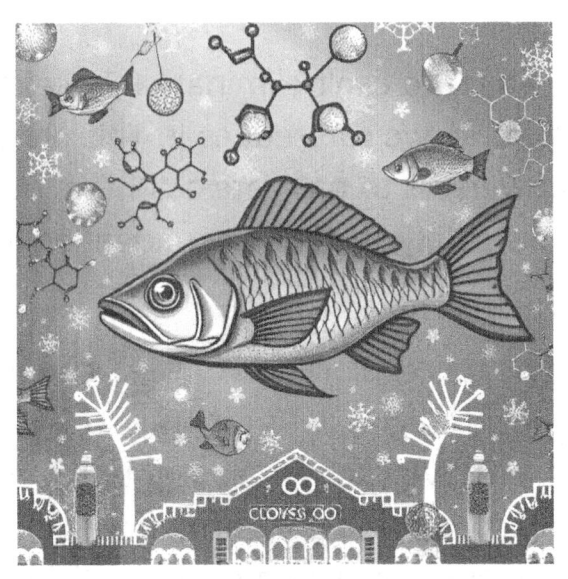

Chapter 13

Bibligraphy

Chapter 1: PFAS: Buck RC, Franklin J, Berger U, Conder JM, Cousins IT, de Voogt P, Jensen AA, Kannan K, Mabury SA, van Leeuwen SP. Perfluoroalkyl and polyfluoroalkyl substances in the environment: terminology, classification, and origins. - Integr Environ Assess Manag. 2011 Oct;7(4):513-41. - Giesy JP, Kannan K. Global distribution of perfluorooctane sulfonate in wildlife. - Environ Sci Technol. 2001 Apr 1;35(7):1339-42. - Lau C,

Anitole K, Hodes C, Lai D, Pfahles-Hutchens A, Seed J. Perfluoroalkyl acids: a review of monitoring and toxicological findings. - Toxicol Sci. 2007 Oct;99(2):366-94. - Bentel MJ, Yu Y, Xu L, Li Z, Wong BM, Men Y, Liu J. Defluorination of Per- and Polyfluoroalkyl Substances (PFASs) with Hydrated Electrons: Structural Dependence and Implications to PFAS Remediation and Management. - Environ Sci Technol. 2019 Mar 19;53(6):3718-3728. - Trier X, Granby K, Christensen JH. Polyfluorinated surfactants (PFS) in paper and board coatings for food packaging. - Environ Sci Pollut Res Int. 2011 Aug;18(7):1108-20 – Chemical Engineering Journal, 2023 – internal documents from 3M and DuPont – Tobacco industry litigation records – Historical records of A.C. Gilbert Company's Atomic Energy Lab

Chapter 2: The History of PFSA: Bibliography: Buck RC, Franklin J, Berger U, et al. Perfluoroalkyl and polyfluoroalkyl substances in the environment: terminology, classification, and origins. - Giesy JP, Kannan K. Global distribution of perfluorooctane sulfonate in wildlife. - Lau C, Anitole K, Hodes C, et al. Perfluoroalkyl acids: a review of monitoring and toxicological findings. - Bentel MJ, Yu Y, Xu L, et al. Defluorination of Per- and Polyfluoroalkyl Substances (PFASs) with Hydrated Electrons: Structural Dependence and Implications to PFAS Remediation and Management. - Trier X, Granby K, Christensen JH. Polyfluorinated surfactants (PFS) in paper and board coatings for food packaging. – Lindstrom, A. B., Strynar, M. J., & Libelo, E. L. (2011). Polyfluorinated compounds: past, present, and future. Environmental Science & Technology, 45(19), 7954-7961. – Grandjean, P., & Clapp, R. (2015). Perfluorinated Alkyl Substances: Emerging Insights Into Health Risks. New Solutions: A Journal of Environmental and Occupational Health Policy, 25(2), 147-163. – Environmental Protection Agency. "PFAS Action Plan." EPA, February 2019. – United States Congress. "National Defense Authorization Act." Various years. – Interstate Technology Regulatory Council. "PFAS Regulations, Guidance, and Advisories." ITRC, Updated regularly, pfas-1.itrcweb.org/fact-sheets/.

Chapter 3: Manufacturers of PFAS: Arkema. "Kynar PVDF Resins." Arkema.com. - BASF. "Fluoropolymers." BASF. com. - Bentel MJ, Yu Y, Xu L, et al. Defluorination of Per- and Polyfluoroalkyl Substances (PFASs) with Hydrated Electrons: Structural Dependence and Implications to PFAS Remediation and Management - Bloomberg Law. "PFAS Makers Face 'Existential Threat' as Liability Concerns Mount." - Buck RC, Franklin J, Berger U, et al. Perfluoroalkyl and polyfluoroalkyl substances in the environment: terminology, classification, and origins - Chemical & Engineering News. "Forever Chemicals: The Dark Side of PFAS." - Corteva Agriscience. "About

Corteva." Corteva.com. - Daikin Chemical. "Fluorochemicals." DaikinChemicals.com. - DuPont de Nemours, Inc. "DuPont Announces Corteva Distribution." DuPont.com. - Environmental Protection Agency. "Basic Information on PFAS." EPA.gov. - Environmental Protection Agency. "Chemours Washington Works History and Safe Drinking Water Act (SWDA) Settlements." - Environmental Protection Agency. "EPA Secures Agreement from Chemours to Conduct New Sampling for PFAS Contamination near Washington Works, WV Facility." - Environmental Protection Agency. "GenX and PFBS Draft Toxicity Assessments." EPA.gov. - Environmental Protection Agency. "PFAS Strategic Roadmap: EPA's Commitments to Action 2021-2024." - Environmental Science & Technology. "Global Emissions of PFAS from 1950 to 2050." - Environmental Working Group. "PFAS Contamination in the U.S." EWG.org. - Giesy JP, Kannan K. Global distribution of perfluorooctane sulfonate in wildlife - Interstate Technology Regulatory Council. "PFAS Technical and Regulatory Guidance Document." ITRC-PFAS.org. - Lau C, Anitole K, Hodes C, et al. Perfluoroalkyl acids: a review of monitoring and toxicological findings - Minnesota Pollution Control Agency. "East Metro | 3M PFAS contamination." - New York State Department of Environmental Conservation. "FACT SHEET Saint-Gobain ~ McCaffrey Street." - Organisation for Economic Co-operation and Development. "Risk Management of Per- and Polyfluoroalkyl Substances (PFASs)." - The Chemours Company. "Our History." Chemours.com. - Trier X, Granby K, Christensen JH. Polyfluorinated surfactants (PFS) in paper and board coatings for food packaging - West Virginia Record. "West Virginia Rivers Coalition sues Chemours over alleged Clean Water Act violations at West Virginia plant."

Chapter 4: PFAS in Our Products and in our Daily Lives: Advanced EMC Technologies. (2024). Why PFAS-Free O-Rings Are the Future of Aerospace and Automotive Engineering - American Chemistry Council. (2024). Fluoropolymers: Essential Materials for Modern Life - Chemical & Engineering News. (2024). The PFAS Dilemma: Balancing Performance and Environmental Impact in Industry - Clariant (2024). PTFE-Free Solutions for Industrial Applications - Clean Production Action (2023). Alternatives to PFAS-Coated Food Packaging - Environmental Protection Agency. (2023). PFAS Strategic Roadmap: EPA's Commitments to Action 2021-2024 - Environmental Science & Technology. (2023). PFAS Migration from Consumer Products to Water Sources: A Comprehensive Review - Glüge, J., et al. (2020). An Overview of the Uses of Per- and Polyfluoroalkyl Substances (PFAS). Environmental Science: Processes & Impacts - Kannan, K., et al. (2017). Occupational Exposure to PFAS in Industrial Settings - National Institute for Occupational Safety and Health (NIOSH). (2024). Workplace Dangers of PFAS "Forever Chemicals" - National Institutes of Health. (2021). Reproductive and Developmental Effects of PFAS - Plastics Engineering Magazine (2023). Tosaf Introduces New Line of PFAS-Free Processing Aids - Schaider, L. A., et al. (2017). Fluorinated Compounds in Cosmetic Products - Susmann, H. P., et al. (2019). PFAS Exposure through Personal Care Products - World Health Organization (2023). PFAS in Drinking Water: Health Concerns and Mitigation Strategies - Z2Data. (2023). Where Are PFAS in Your Electronics Supply Chain?

Chapter 5: PFAS Contamination from Industry, Manufactures, Landfills, and Agriculture: Ahrens, L., et al. (2016). Environmental Science & Technology. - Bentel MJ, Yu Y, Xu L, et al. Defluorination of Per- and Polyfluoroalkyl Substances (PFASs) with Hydrated Electrons: Structural Dependence and Implications to PFAS Remediation and Management. - Buck RC, Franklin J, Berger U, et al. Perfluoroalkyl and polyfluoroalkyl substances in the environment: terminology, classification, and origins. - Carey, M. (2022). Fatal Fertilizer: PFAS Contamination of Farmland from Biosolids and Potential Federal Solutions. Pace Environmental Law Review. - Chen, X., et al. (2020). Environmental Science & Technology. - Environmental Working Group. (2022). EWG.org. - Environmental Working Group. (2024). PFAS in Agriculture:

A Growing Concern. - Giesy JP, Kannan K. Global distribution of perfluorooctane sulfonate in wildlife. - Glüge J, Scheringer M, Cousins IT, et al. An overview of the uses of per- and polyfluoroalkyl substances (PFAS). - Hamid, H., & Li, L. (2016). Ecocycles. - Lang, J. R., et al. (2016). Environmental Science & Technology. - Lau C, Anitole K, Hodes C, et al. Perfluoroalkyl acids: a review of monitoring and toxicological findings. - Maine Department of Agriculture, Conservation and Forestry. (2025). PFAS Assistance for Maine Farmers. - Maine Department of Environmental Protection. (2025). PFAS Contamination Report. - National Farmers Union. (2025). The PFAS Crisis in American Agriculture: A Call to Action. - Pillsbury Law. (2024). New Lawsuit shows PFAS Exposure for Fertilizer Manufacturers. - Santen M, Kallee U. Chemistry for any weather: Greenpeace tests outdoor clothes for perfluorinated toxins. - Stone, F. (2023). The Fall of a Family Farm: PFAS and the Dairy Industry. - The Toxic Legacy: PFAS Contamination and the Agricultural Crisis. - Trier X, Granby K, Christensen JH. Polyfluorinated surfactants (PFS) in paper and board coatings for food packaging. - U.S. Department of Agriculture. (2025). Per-and Polyfluoroalkyl Substances FAQ. - U.S. Environmental Protection Agency. (2021). EPA.gov. - U.S. Environmental Protection Agency. (2024). EPA Awards $15 Million for Research on PFAS Exposure and Reduction in Agriculture. - U.S. Environmental Protection Agency.

(2024). PFAS in Food: Current Understanding and Future Directions. - Venkatesan, A.K., & Halden, R.U. (2013). Water Research. - Wang, Z., et al. (2022). Environmental Science & Technology.\

CHapter 6: The PFAS Nightmare: DuPont's Toxic Legacy in Parkersburg; Lyons, - C. (2007). Stain-Resistant, Non-stick, Waterproof, and Lethal: The Hidden Dangers of C8. Praeger Publishers - Rich, N. (2016). "The Lawyer Who Became DuPont's Worst Nightmare." The New York Times Magazine - Lerner, S. (2015). "The Teflon Toxin." The Intercept - Hawthorne, M. (2019). "DuPont, Chemours Agree to Pay $670 Million to Settle PFOA Lawsuits." Chicago Tribune - U.S. Environmental Protection Agency. (2021). "PFOA, PFOS and Other PFASs" - Bilott, R. (2019). Exposure: Poisoned Water, Corporate Greed, and One Lawyer's Twenty-Year Battle against DuPont. Atria Books - C8 Science Panel. (2012). "C8 Probable Link Reports" - Ohio Attorney General's Office. (2023). "DuPont Settlement Press Release" - Halpern, M. (2015). "How DuPont Concealed the Dangers of the New Teflon Toxin." Scientific American - Emmett, E. A., et al. (2006). "Community Exposure to Perfluorooctanoate: Relationships Between Serum Concentrations and Exposure Sources." Journal of Occupational and Environmental Medicine - Tillett, T. (2007). "Serum PFOA Levels in Residents of Communities Near a Teflon Production Facility." Environmental Health Perspectives - C8 Health Project. (2009). "Design, Methods, and Participants." Environmental Health Perspectives - PFAS Project Lab. (2019). "Parkersburg, West Virginia." The PFAS Project Lab - Governor Mike DeWine and Ohio Attorney General Dave Yost. (2023). "State Secures $110 Million Settlement with DuPont for Environmental Restoration Along Ohio River." Office of the Governor of Ohio - Leach v. E.I. du Pont de Nemours & Co., et al. (2001). Case Documents Summary on PFOA Contaminat

Chapter 7: PFAS and Human Health: – Agency for Toxic Substances and Disease Registry (2024). Human Exposure: PFAS Information for Clinicians - Environmental Working Group (2023). Groundbreaking Map Shows Toxic 'Forever Chemicals' - National Institute of Environmental Health Sciences (2024). Perfluoroalkyl and Polyfluoroalkyl Substances (PFAS) - Johansson et al., Animal Studies on Neurodevelopmental Effects of PFAS (2009-2013) - Nature Journal (2024). Revisiting the "Forever Chemicals": PFOA and PFOS Exposure in Global Water Systems - Guelfo JL, Adamson DT. Evaluation of a national data set for insights into sources, composition, and concentrations of per- and polyfluoroalkyl substances (PFASs) in U.S. drinking water. Environmental Pollution, 236:505-513 - Adamson, David T., et al. (2020). Mass-Based, Field-Scale Demonstration of PFAS

Retention within AFFF-Associated Source Areas. Environmental Science & Technology, 54(24):15768–15777 - Environmental Working Group (2020). PFAS Contamination of Drinking Water Far More Prevalent Than Reported by EPA - EWG Tap Water Database (2024). PFAS in Drinking Water: A National Crisis.

Chapter 8: Wildlife, Birds, Fish Fisherman and Hunters : 2023 Environmental Working Group (EWG) National Freshwater Fish PFAS Study - 2024 New York State Department of Environmental Conservation Seneca Lake Fish Tissue Analysis - Minnesota Department of Health PFAS Fish Consumption Guidelines - Chesapeake Bay Program PCB Contamination Report - Waterkeeper Alliance 2024 PFAS in U.S. Surface Water Study - North Carolina Department of Environmental Quality Cape Fear River Fish Consumption Advisories - Environmental Working Group (EWG) Great Lakes PFAS Contamination Analysis - United States Geological Survey (USGS) National Water Quality Assessment of PFAS in Groundwater - Michigan Department of Health and Human Services Lake Superior Smelt PFAS Investigation - Georgia Environmental Protection Division Conasauga River PFAS Data Report - U.S. Department of Defense PFAS Contamination at Military Installations Report - 2024 Maine Department of Inland Fisheries and Wildlife PFAS Deer Consumption Advisories - Czech University of Life Sciences Wild Boar Liver PFAS Study - New Mexico Environment Department Holloman Air Force Base Lake PFAS Report - Iowa Department of Natural Resources Upland Game Bird Contaminant Data - Michigan Department of Environment, Great Lakes, and Energy Clark's Marsh Deer PFAS Analysis - European Food Safety Authority PFAS Regulations and Risk Assessment - Victoria Environmental Protection Authority Gippsland Lakes Waterfowl PFAS Testing Program

Chapter 9: Regulations: U.S. Environmental Protection Agency, "National Primary Drinking Water Regulations for PFAS" (April 10, 2024) - U.S. Environmental Protection Agency, "PFOA and PFOS Designation as Hazardous Substances under CERCLA" (April 19, 2024) - U.S. Environmental Protection Agency, "PFAS Enforcement Discretion and Settlement Policy Under CERCLA" (April 19, 2024) - European Union, "Comprehensive Ban on Non-Essential PFAS Uses" (February 2023) - Australian Industrial Chemicals Introduction Scheme, "Regulatory Measures for PFOA and Related Compounds" (2023) - Minnesota Department of Health, "PFAS Ban in Consumer Products" (2025) - U.S. Environmental Protection Agency, "PFAS Strategic Roadmap" (November 2024) - Stockholm Convention on Persistent Organic Pollutants, "Framework for Eliminating or Reducing Persistent Organic Pollutants" (2022) - U.S. Department of

Defense, "PFAS Actions for Defense Personnel and Installations" (2024) - Environment and Climate Change Canada, "PFAS Regulations in Canada" (2024) - United Kingdom Health and Safety Executive, "Regulatory Management Options for PFAS" (202

Chapter 10: PFSA Litigation: Environmental Protection Agency, "PFOA and PFOS Designation as Hazardous Substances under CERCLA" (April 2024) - 3M Company, "PFAS Settlement with Public Water Systems" (2024) - Tyco Fire Products, "Settlement for Water Contamination from Firefighting Foam" (April 2024) - BASF, "Settlement with U.S. Public Water Systems over PFAS Contamination" (May 2024) - Carrier Global Corporation, "Resolution of Firefighting Foam Claims" (October 2024) - New York State Supreme Court, "Hoosick Falls PFAS Contamination Settlement" (2021) - U.S. District Court for the Southern District of Ohio, "DuPont Parkersburg PFAS Settlement" (2017) - Nantucket Superior Court, "Class Action against DuPont, 3M, and BASF" (November 2024) - New York State Supreme Court, "Firefighter Ulcerative Colitis Case" (October 2024) - U.S. District Court for the District of New Jersey, "Kenvue/J&J Band-Aid PFAS Class Action" (July 2024) - U.S. District Court for the Northern District of California, "Bic Razors PFAS Claims" (May 2024) - Minnesota Attorney General's Office, "3M PFAS Settlement" (2018) - Texas Attorney General's Office,

"Lawsuit against PFAS Manufacturers" (December 2024) - Maryland Attorney General's Office, "Expanded Claims against Carrier Fire Americas" (November 2024) - Illinois Attorney General's Office, "PFAS Lawsuit against 3M and Others" (2024) - Alabama Attorney General's Office, "PFAS Lawsuit against 3M and Others" (2024) - Minnesota Legislature, "PFAS Ban on Consumer Products" (2025) - European Commission, "Proposal for Comprehensive Ban on Non-Essential PFAS Uses" (February 2023) - UK Health and Safety Executive, "PFAS Restriction Proposal" (2024) - Japan Ministry of Health, Labour and Welfare, "PFAS Limits in Drinking Water" (2023) - Environment and Climate Change Canada, "PFAS Regulations" (2024) - Quebec Ministry of Environment and Climate Change, "PFAS Standards" (2024)

Chapter 11: PFAS in Fresh Produce: Environmental Working Group, "PFAS in Food Packaging: What's in Your Takeout?" (2020) - Dow Chemical Company, "Safety Data Sheet: Fluroxypyr" (2021) - BASF, "Clopyralid Technical Fact Sheet" (2019) - Environmental Protection Agency, "PFAS in Biosolids" (2021) - Food and Drug Administration, "Analytical Results for PFAS in 2022 Total Diet Study" (2022) - Journal of Agricultural and Food Chemistry, "Uptake of Per- and Polyfluoroalkyl Substances by Plants" (2020) - Environmental Science & Technology, "PFAS in Imported Produce: A Growing Concern" (2021)

- Consumer Reports, "PFAS in Food Packaging: A Market Survey" (2022) - Nature Food, "Global Assessment of PFAS Contamination in Agricultural Soils" (2021) - Environmental Health Perspectives, "PFAS Migration from Food Contact Materials" (2020)

Chapter 12: So What Can We Do ? Grandjean, P., & Landrigan, P. J. (2014). Neurobehavioural effects of developmental toxicity. The Lancet Neurology, 13(3), 330-338. - Hu, X. C., Andrews, D. Q., Lindstrom, A. B., Bruton, T. A., Schaider, L. A., Grandjean, P., ... & Sunderland, E. M. (2016). Detection of poly-and perfluoroalkyl substances (PFASs) in US drinking water linked to industrial sites, military fire training areas, and wastewater treatment plants. Environmental Science & Technology Letters, 3(10), 344-350. - Karásková, P., Venier, M., Melymuk, L., Bečanová, J., Vojta, Š., Prokeš, R., ... & Klánová, J. (2016). Perfluorinated alkyl substances (PFASs) in household dust in Central Europe and North America. Environment International, 94, 315-324. - Kotthoff, M., Müller, J., Jürling, H., Schlummer, M., & Fiedler, D. (2015). Perfluoroalkyl and polyfluoroalkyl substances in consumer products. Environmental Science and Pollution Research, 22(19), 14546-14559. - Sunderland, E. M., Hu, X. C., Dassuncao, C., Tokranov, A. K., Wagner, C. C., & Allen, J. G. (2019). A review of the pathways of human exposure to poly-and perfluoroalkyl substances

(PFASs) and present understanding of health effects. Journal of Exposure Science & Environmental Epidemiology, 29(2), 131-147.

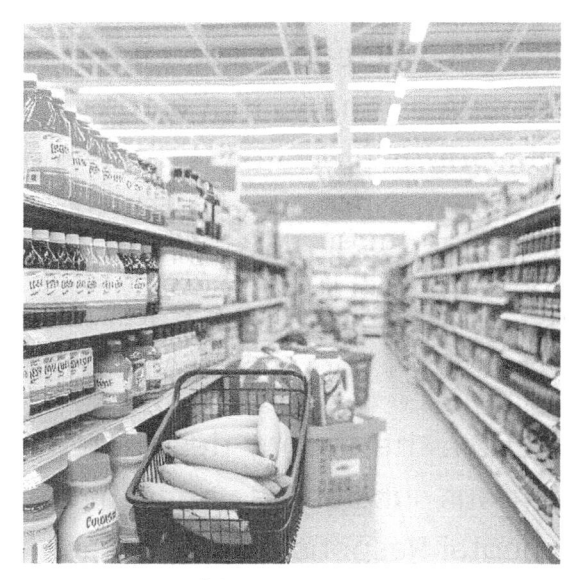

Chapter 14

EPA Update 2025

On April 10, 2024, the U.S. Environmental Protection Agency (EPA) finalized national primary drinking water regulations for six PFAS chemical compounds. The new standards set maximum contaminant levels (MCLs) of 4 parts per trillion (ppt) for PFOA and PFOS. For PFNA, PFHxS, PFBS, and GenX chemicals, the EPA established a hazard index limit to address the combined effects of these PFAS.

These regulations, a significant milestone in environmental health, mandate public water systems to monitor for the six PFAS and reduce levels if they exceed the standards. The EPA estimates that 6-10% of the 66,000 regulated public drinking water systems may have to take action to reduce PFAS levels. This rule marks a significant step in addressing PFAS contamination in drinking water across the United States. The EPA also took action regarding cleanup of PFAS contamination.

On April 19, 2024, the agency designated PFOA and PFOS as hazardous substances under the Comprehensive Environmental Response, Compensation, and Liability Act (CERCLA), also known as Superfund. This designation allows the EPA to require responsible parties to clean up contaminated sites and reimburse the government for EPA-led cleanups.

The same day, the EPA released its PFAS Enforcement Discretion and Settlement Policy under CERCLA, guiding how the agency will approach enforcement and settlement negotiations related to PFAS contamination. The European Union has taken significant steps to address PFAS pollution. In February 2023, the EU announced a comprehensive ban on all non-essential uses of PFAS, covering about 10,000 compounds. This wide-ranging restriction aims to phase out PFAS in various products, including food packaging, cosmetics, and textiles, demonstrating a proactive approach to environmental health. The ban is expected to take effect in 2026, allowing industries time to adapt and find alternatives. Australia has also implemented regulatory measures, with the Industrial Chemicals Introduction Scheme (AICIS) introducing new requirements for PFOA and related compounds in 2023.

The ban is expected to take effect in 2026, allowing industries time to adapt and find alternatives. Australia has also implemented regulatory measures, with the Industrial Chemicals Introduction Scheme (AICIS) introducing new requirements for PFOA and related compounds in 2023.

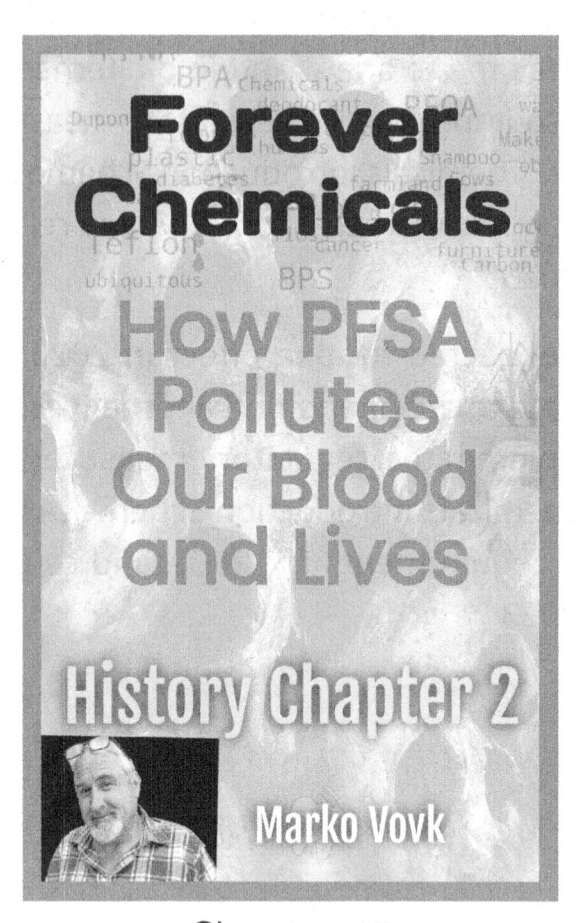

Chapter 15

Further Reading

Hey there! I'm thrilled to share my journey into book publishing with you. After semi-retiring and weathering the storm of COVID-19, I've discovered a new passion that's set my creative spirit on fire! Now, I'll be the first to admit I'm no English major or fiction virtuoso. But what I lack in literary prowess, I make up for with a treasure trove of education, knowledge, and real-world experiences. Plus, I've got research skills that would make a detective jealous!

Each book I craft is a labor of love, penned by you honestly, with a bit of help from some nifty editing software. I even design my covers—talk about wearing multiple hats! Regarding publishing, I'm proudly independent, embracing the self-publishing route.

I will tell you a secret: my writing has been quite the journey. With each book, I feel like I'm leveling up and honing my craft. While I may not be gunning for a spot on The New York Times bestseller list (yet!), my books are bursting at the seams with information.

Here's the beauty of my books – you can dive in from any chapter and still strike gold. Fair warning, though: I pack in information like I'm preparing for an intellectual apocalypse. And yes, my experiences and beliefs might color the pages a bit. But hey, that's what makes them uniquely mine.

I always encourage my readers to treat my books as a springboard for exploration. Dive deeper, question everything, and forge your path to the truth. Sometimes, I might get a tad carried away and exaggerate a concept or two—it's all part of my charm! I'm eager to hear from my readers. Do you have suggestions or ideas for improvements? Please shoot me an email! Thanks to the magic of Amazon KDP, I can tweak and update faster than you can say "revised edition."

As we wrap up 2024, I'm proud to look back at the books I've published over the past two years. It's been a wild ride, and I can't wait to see what literary adventures await in the coming year! Remember, if you're looking for a no-nonsense, information-packed read with a dash of personal flair, you've come to the right place. Happy reading, and here's to the joy of lifelong learning!

1. Avoid Waterproofing, Drain Cleaning and Foundation Repair Scams

2. Childless Cat Lady: Movement, Dynamics, Health, and Political Influence

3. Make Your Home Great Again

4. Deep Down The Rabbit Hole Poetry

5. Don't Rent this Home, Condo, or Apartment

6. Nuclear Extinction Event Is Killing Our Families

7. Pets: The Hidden Costs of Companionship

8. Project 2025 Quick Review

9. The Water You Drink May Be Killing You

10. Fix Your Toxic Home and Liver Longer

11. Make Your Home Great Again

Made in the USA
Monee, IL
13 March 2025